♥ Praise for "What Does That LGBTQIA+ Label Mean?" ♥

"Even if you think you know what it means to be gay, you'll learn and be amused by so much more in *What Does That LGBTQIA+ Label Mean?*"

— **Jim Obergefell,** civil rights activist and named plaintiff in the landmark Supreme Court marriage equality case Obergefell v. Hodges, which legalized same-sex marriage in the United States

"Everyone deserves their own oasis."

— **Lamarr Houston,** former American football outside linebacker, eight-year NFL veteran, and League Ventures Founder

"Take it from Edie, it's not just the bisexuals who are greedy <wink>."

— **Judith Kasen-Windsor,** surviving spouse of Edie Windsor (United States v. Windsor) public speaker, philanthropist, & LGBTQ+ activist and advocate

"As a Marine veteran of the Iraq War and an openly gay man whose colleagues risked their lives to save mine, I can tell you that being gay, lesbian, bisexual, or transgender does not damage unit cohesion. Books like *What Does That LGBTQIA+ Label Mean?* help us to break the binary of gender and sexuality so we can come to realize that we're all equally valuable and deserving of equitable opportunity to live our lives to the fullest."

— **Retired Marine Staff Sergeant Eric Alva,** the first American soldier injured in the Iraq War, LGBTQ rights advocate and author

"Fiona's important voice from within the bi+ community is loud and clear in *What Does That LGBTQIA+ Label Mean?*"

— **Robyn Ochs,** speaker, writer, activist on LGBTQ issues and a challenger of false binaries

"In *What Does That LGBTQIA+ Label Mean?,* Fiona reaches inside and out to connect people to their own experiences and those of others. At PFLAG, we meet people where they are and bring them along; Fiona's book takes that approach in her own beautifully unique and totally enjoyable way."

— **Diego Miguel Sanchez,** APR, Director of Advocacy, Policy, and Partnerships, PFLAG National

"Fiona's voice in *What Does That LGBTQIA+ Label Mean?* is the fierce yet friendly advocate LGBTQ+ kids need."

— **Judy and Dennis Shepard,** human rights advocates and parents of Matthew Shepard

"A delightful and insightful primer on all things LGBTQ. I'd say it's tongue-in-cheek ... but perhaps I've confused my anatomy."

— **Annise D. Parker,** CEO, Victory Fund and 61st Mayor of Houston, Texas

"*What Does That LGBTQIA+ Label Mean?* is a witty, often hilarious, and much needed guide to being LGBTQ that families around the world will come to rely on and treasure."

— **Jake and Hannah Graf,** award-winning actor, MBE retired British Army Officer, and "The UK's most influential LGBT Power Couple" — The Guardian

"Fiona's own vulnerability in *What Does That LGBTQIA+ Label Mean?* makes her LGBTQ+ explainers all the more relatable."

— **Ellen Kahn,** Senior Director, Programs and Partnerships, Human Rights Campaign

"The main thing I found that Fiona has straight in *What Does That LGBTQIA+ Label Mean?* are her facts. Top those off with her honesty and openness, this is a great read."

— **Andrew Reynolds,** Senior Research Scholar, Princeton University and author of many books including "*The Children of Harvey Milk: How LGBTQ Politicians Changed the World*" (Oxford, 2018)

"As a longtime Bi ally, this is exactly the kind of book I've been waiting for. As our culture continues to get beyond the binary we still see far too much stereotyping and misinformation about the largest part of our LGBT community. Fiona's approach of making conversation and education accessible and fun will go a long way. My hope is that this book ends up in the hands of all the folks who need it, in the LGBT community and larger culture."

— **Cathy Renna,** Communications Director, National LGBTQ Task Force

"*What Does That LGBTQIA+ Label Mean?* is an artistic and humorous primer on the perpetually contested nature of bisexual identity."

— **Zackary Drucker,** artist and filmmaker

"Fiona is a gifted and experienced storyteller who humanizes real world issues in ways that enlighten and showcase the common humanity we all share. At a time when more attention and understanding need to happen around LGBTQ issues, Fiona's magnetic personality, refreshing approach to educating, and visibility as a bi woman add unique and necessary elements to the media at large."

— **Sarah Kate Ellis,** President and CEO, GLAAD

"This book is perfect for allies and advocates looking for clear answers to what some see as the challenging topics of gender, identity, and sexuality. Fiona brings her charm and wit to the pages as she addresses each subject with clarity and compassion through engaging storytelling. The reader will even find answers to questions they didn't know they needed to be able to answer."

— **Amanda Simpson,** Aerospace Executive and Transgender Pioneer

"Fiona's perspective and stories kept my imagination engaged in an otherwise hard to deliver subject. I giggled at times and shed tears at others after seeing parts of myself represented properly in a work without using compromising terms or ambiguous keynotes you hear from every talk about sex, gender, and sexuality. I will be recommending this to others and have added it to my collection of resources."

— **Lilith Kidd,** United States Marine Corps combat veteran and LGBTQIA+ advocate

"*What Does That LGBTQIA+ Label Mean?* is irreverent, fun, and simply delightful. Fiona approaches topics that are often off limits with honesty, vulnerability, and panache. She breaks down the bits and bobbles of the 'Alphabet Mafia' with a sultry gentility that makes me grin from ear to ear. Whether you are learning a whole new language around queerness, or a seasoned member of our beloved community, there is something informative and endearing about how Fiona moves through her own journey and the queer lexicon."

— **Dalila Ali Rajah,** Out bisexual actress, writer, *art*ivist, Mom, and founder of Black Queer Joy

"*What Does That LGBTQIA+ Label Mean?* is an absolute delight, and a much needed addition to literature on the largest, and often misunderstood, part of the LGBT community. A common sense explainer for many of the most frequently asked questions about queer people, it is filled with Fiona's wicked sense of humor and experience from working to advance the interests of people across the LGBT spectrum over 20 years."

— **Brynn Tannehill,** author of *Everything You Ever Wanted to Know About Trans* (*But Were Afraid to Ask)*

"When my daughter Avery began her transition in 2011, the information I found was very binary and didn't prepare a parent new to LGBTQ+ topics like myself to understand gender and sexuality differences. It can be intimidating! Thankfully we now have *What Does That LGBTQIA+ Label Mean?* With compassion and humor, Fiona has created an easy and direct read for parents wanting to understand their kids' LGBTQ+ identities. Definitely have this book at home over the holidays."

— **Debi Jackson,** the self-described "conservative Southern Baptist Republican from Alabama" now speaking on behalf of transgender children and their families around the world

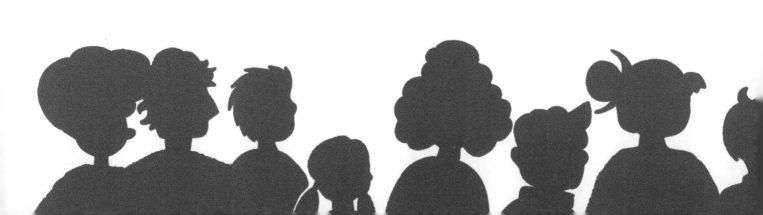

What Does That LGBTQIA+ Label Mean?

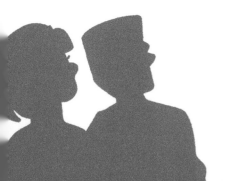

What Does That LGBTQIA+ Label Mean?

Explaining the Spectrum of Gender and Sexuality with Humor and Ease

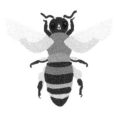

FIONA DAWSON (SHE/HER)

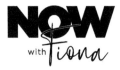
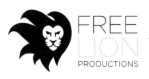

Edited by: August Li (he/him),
Lisa Canfield (she/her), Lori McFerran (she/her)

Illustrated by: Syd Cordoba (they/them)
Cover design by: Cornelia Murariu (she/her)
Typeset by: Cornelia Murariu (she/her)

For permission requests, write to the publisher, addressed "Attention: Permissions Coordinator," at the address below.

Publish Your Purpose
141 Weston Street, #155
Hartford, CT, 06141

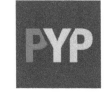

The opinions expressed by the Author are not necessarily those held by Publish Your Purpose.

Ordering Information: Quantity sales and special discounts are available on quantity purchases by corporations, associations, and others. For details, contact the publisher at hello@publishyourpurpose.com.

Printed in the United States of America.
ISBN: 979-8-88797-991-5 (hardcover)
ISBN: 979-8-88797-990-8 (paperback)
ISBN: 979-8-88797-118-6 (ebook)

Library of Congress Control Number:
2024904987

Second edition, April 2024

The information contained within this book is strictly for informational purposes. The material may include information, products, or services by third parties. As such, the Author and Publisher do not assume responsibility or liability for any third-party material or opinions. The publisher is not responsible for websites (or their content) that are not owned by the publisher. Readers are advised to do their own due diligence when it comes to making decisions.

The mission of Publish Your Purpose is to discover and publish authors who are striving to make a difference in the world. We give underrepresented voices power and a stage to share their stories, speak their truth, and impact their communities. Do you have a book idea you would like us to consider publishing? Please visit PublishYourPurpose.com for more information.

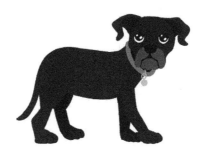

♥ This beautiful pitbull-boxer mix is Ms. Maizie Rai #TheAdventuresOfMaizieRai. ♥

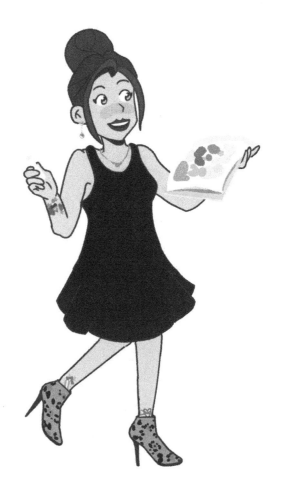

♥ Fiona ♥

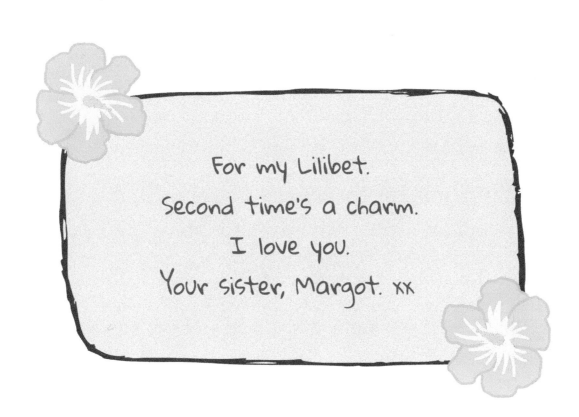

For my Lilibet.
Second time's a charm.
I love you.
Your sister, Margot. xx

CONTENTS

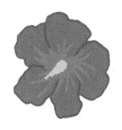

Foreword   xvii

Introduction: What's All the Fuss about These Labels Anyway?   xxi

1. What's the Difference between "Cisgender" and "Transgender?"   1
2. Is Being Transgender the Same as Being Gay?   5
3. How Do I Know What My Gender Is?   7
4. What's the "QIA" in "LGBTQIA"?   9
5. What Does the Word "Queer" Mean?   13
6. What Does It Mean to Be Intersex?   17
7. What Do You Mean Some People Don't Want to Have Sexual Relations?   19
8. Do Transgender Men Actually Exist?   23
9. Is Being Nonbinary Just Cool These Days?   27
10. Are Drag Queens Transgender?   31
11. Are Bisexuals Just Greedy?   35
12. Which Label Is Better, Bisexual or Pansexual?   37
13. Why Are We Saying, "Hey Guys!" to Greet Women?   41
14. If a Straight Man Wants to Make Love with a Transgender Woman, Does It Mean He's Gay?   45
15. Do All Transgender Men Want Male Genitalia?   47
16. How do Transgender Women Pee in a Public Restroom?   51
17. Why Does Allowing Athletes who are Transgender to Compete in School Sports Make America Great?   55
18. Why Can't I Love the Sinner but Hate the Sin?   59
19. Why Are Straight People Putting Their Pronouns on Zoom?   63
20. How Can You Use "They" for One Person if It's a Plural Word?   67
21. How Can I Keep My Kids Safe from Transgender and Gay People?   71

Conclusion: How Can I Be the Best Ally Ever?!   75

Acknowledgments   79

Additional Resources   83

Bibliography   87

Afterword   93

About the Author   95

About the Illustrator   97

Work with Fiona   99

A CHEAT SHEET TO QUICKLY FIND WHAT YOU'RE LOOKING FOR ...

I realize that the chapter titles in this book may not indicate the actual core messages in the text. So if Uncle Tedd pops off at dinner one night that he heard the term "gender dysphoria" on the news, and he's got no bloody idea what that means, you can quickly glance down the column on the right, find "gender dysphoria," and have him read the chapter lined up on the left before dessert is served. For a more comprehensive dictionary style of definitions, check out the resources listed in the "MORE LGBTQIA+ LANGUAGE THINGS TO KNOW" section towards the end of this book.

	CHEEKY CHAPTER TITLE	TOPICS THAT ARE ACTUALLY COVERED
	Introduction: What's All the Fuss about These Labels Anyway?	Change happens · Self-awareness · Awareness of others · Love
1	What's the Difference between "Cisgender" and "Transgender?"	Cisgender · Transgender · Biological Sex vs. Gender
2	Is Being Transgender the Same as Being Gay?	Transgender · Gay · Intersex · Gender · Biological Sex · Sexual orientation · Gender vs. Attraction
3	How Do I Know What My Gender Is?	Gender is 1) Who you know yourself to be, 2) How you express yourself to the world, and 3) How the world sees you · Biological Sex vs. Gender · Assignment at birth · SAAB · AFAB · AMAB
4	What's the "QIA" in "LGBTQIA"?	Lesbian · Gay · Bisexual · Pansexual · Transgender · Trans* · Nonbinary · Queer · Questioning · Intersex · Asexual · Aromatic · Two-Spirit · Heterosexual
5	What Does the Word "Queer" Mean?	Lesbian · Gay · Bisexual · Transgender · Queer · Gender · Sexual orientation
6	What Does It Mean to Be Intersex?	Intersex · Chromosomes · Genitals · Reproductive tissue
7	What Do You Mean Some People Don't Want to Have Sexual Relations?	Asexual · Attraction is: 1) Love, 2) Romance, and 3) Sex
8	Do Transgender Men Actually Exist?	Puberty blockers · Physical/medical transition ·
9	Is Being Nonbinary Just Cool These Days?	Nonbinary · Two-Spirit · History of language ·

	CHEEKY CHAPTER TITLE	TOPICS THAT ARE ACTUALLY COVERED
10	Are Drag Queens Transgender?	Drag queens/drag · Gay · Sexual orientation vs. Gender identity/ expression · Spectrums
11	Are Bisexuals Just Greedy?	Sexual orientation is: 1) Attraction, 2) Identity, and 3) Behavior
12	Which Label Is Better, Bisexual or Pansexual?	Fluidity of Sexual orientation · Bisexual · Pansexual
13	Why Are We Saying, "Hey Guys!" to Greet Women?	Gendered language · Origin of "guys" · History of language
14	If a Straight Man Wants to Make Love with a Transgender Woman, Does It Mean He's Gay?	Sexual orientation is: 1) Attraction, 2) Identity, and 3) Behavior · Sex tissue vs. Brain matter
15	Do All Transgender Men Want Male Genitalia?	Physical/medical transition · Intersex · Gender dysphoria · Prosthetics
16	How do Transgender Women Pee in a Public Restroom?	Gender vs. Biological Sex · Stand To Pee · Gender expression
17	Why Does Allowing Athletes who are Transgender to Compete in School Sports Make America Great?	Existence of trans* people · Biology vs. Stereotypes · Human variance · The Olympics · Medical transition · Importance of sports · Segregation
18	Why Can't I Love the Sinner but Hate the Sin?	The Bible · History of language · Love
19	Why Are Straight People Putting Their Pronouns on Zoom?	Being misgendered · Social construct of gender
20	How Can You Use "They" for One Person if It's a Plural Word?	History of language · Social construct of gender · Implicit bias
21	How Can I Keep My Kids Safe from Transgender and Gay People?	Domestic and sexual violence · Violent crime · Media bias · Gender identity and Sexual orientation · Prevalence of LGBTQIA+ youth
	Conclusion: How Can I Be the Best Ally Ever?!	Know yourself · Consider others · Be kind · Be courageous · Love

"We want a world where boys can feel, girls can lead, and the rest of us can not only exist but thrive. This is not about erasing men and women but rather acknowledging that man and woman are two of many stars in a constellation that do not compete but amplify one another's shine."

—Alok Vaid-Menon,
Beyond the Gender Binary [1]

Foreword

By Laila Ireland (She/her),
Army Veteran and
LGBTQIA+ Advocate

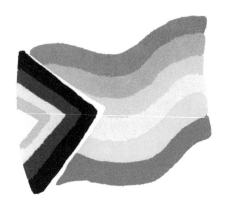

To be close to Fiona Dawson is to have hit the lottery of friendships.

Picture this: It is seven in the morning on March 23, 2013 in San Antonio, Texas. The air is crisp and chilly, and smells of freshly cut grass swimming through the ever so light breeze. As I pull on my black and scratchy cardigan I look out my kitchen window and think to myself, "Am I really ready for what I am about to do?" I had been virtually connected with Fiona through a mutual friend and set up an in-person meeting with her just to formally introduce ourselves to see if my own story would benefit the *TransMilitary* project she was working on.

I made the ten minute drive down the road from my house to meet with her. I parked my truck and made my way to the lobby of the Aloft hotel. When I walked in, I noticed three things: the tiny corner cafe brewing fresh coffee, three empty mustard yellow bar stools sitting quietly at the wooden bar top table, and the abstract art that lined the walls. I later realized that all three of these things reflected what was

happening in that present moment. I reached for my cell phone to send Fiona a message that I had arrived and was waiting in the lobby. I positioned myself on one of the mustard yellow bar stools that stood in direct view of the elevator. It was surprisingly soft and comfortable. A few minutes went by and the elevator bell dinged. For a moment, my heart beat dramatically in my chest. For a moment, I wanted to run. For a moment, I felt I had made a mistake. The elevator doors open and out walks this short woman with a red pixie cut and a smile of a million diamonds. She wore a red sheer scarf placed neatly around her neck draping over a black long sleeve blouse, and distressed jeans completed with a brown belt and boots. I immediately felt that this woman had an energy so captivating it makes it almost impossible to pull away from her.

I quickly stood to meet Fiona and we exchanged a hug that felt like we had known one another our whole lives. I motioned to the coffee counter and she said in her cute British accent,

"Oh bless you, I need this to start my day." We returned to the bar stools to sit and we talked about her vision for *TransMilitary*. I knew that in order to participate and share my story publicly on camera I was going to have to be more vulnerable than I ever had been before in my life. There were moments during our conversation when I wanted to run from the potential public exposure and where I thought I'd made a mistake in considering being a part of her project. But Fiona's authentic compassion, respectful curiosity, and own willingness to be vulnerable made me know that I needn't worry. There was just something so genuine about Fiona and her passion that made me feel extremely comfortable. Comfortable enough to divulge intimate details about my life that would later become a catalyst to the bigger vision she had, and an even bigger tool for what was coming. And in that moment, I knew that our friendship, partnership, and work were just about to begin their long and incredible journey. As we departed I realized the coffee resembled our brewing sisterhood, the chairs reflected the comfort and ease brought about by understanding Fiona's vision and being able to open up about intimate details about my life, and I personally related to being like the art that lined the walls of the hotel lobby. Just like that art, I felt seen even though I was different. I felt beautiful. I felt valued.

What Does That LGBTQIA+ Label Mean? is going to help others not just peer into the windows of a world they may know nothing about, but land them into the stories themselves to help each person navigate the understanding of it all. On many occasions, I have witnessed Fiona ask gentle but thought-provoking questions that force her subjects to really do their best to understand their own stories. She helps people construct their own narrative in a way that lets the audience feel the moment's emotions and see the story from the storyteller's perspective. Fiona's writing and storytelling technique, in all forms of media she embraces from books to films, truly helps move hearts and minds to a place of better understanding and vital self reflection.

My experiences and relationship with Fiona have helped me use my own story as a tool to help others find their voice. With everything I have learned from and with Fiona, I have been able to help others begin their own journeys to find, embrace, and celebrate their true, authentic selves in a patriarch-driven world that constantly is telling us that we are different from the societal norm. It's about being brave enough to face the world and share it out loud, and with pride.

Fiona's vision and work have been monumentally impactful. If it weren't for her hard work and dedication to her vision, my husband, Logan, and my story originally told in her short New York Times op-doc *Transgender, at War and in Love*, would not have made it to national platforms. Like that time Logan and I ended up on The Ellen DeGeneres Show. Or that time we made the centerfold story of People Magazine. Or that time we got to walk the red (it was actually blue) carpet of the MTV Video Music Awards. Or when Logan and I attended the Obama White House Pride Reception as the very first openly transgender couple invited while both actively serving in the United States military. Or even that time we were able to use our stories to change a long-standing military policy that would acknowledge and allow transgender troops to serve openly in the United States military. These are just a few of the incredible moments resulting in the work Fiona has done.

While many people may feel that having someone else tell their story—especially a white, cisgender person—might not align with their vision and takes away from their authenticity, Fiona does the exact opposite. In her work, she helps you shape your story to make it easier for everyone to understand. She doesn't take away the power of you telling your own story, she helps you enhance your power. From here I only see Fiona's media platform continue to grow to where she helps empower even more people to do just that—tell their stories from their perspective. Authentically. With power and pride. This book is another stepping stone to get there. My hope is that with this book, she changes more lives like she has mine.

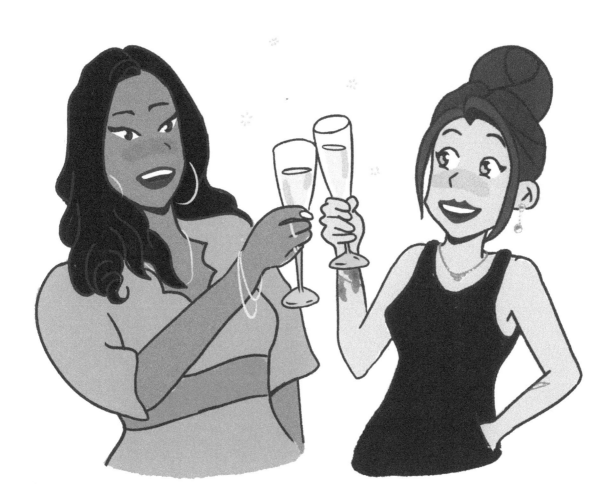

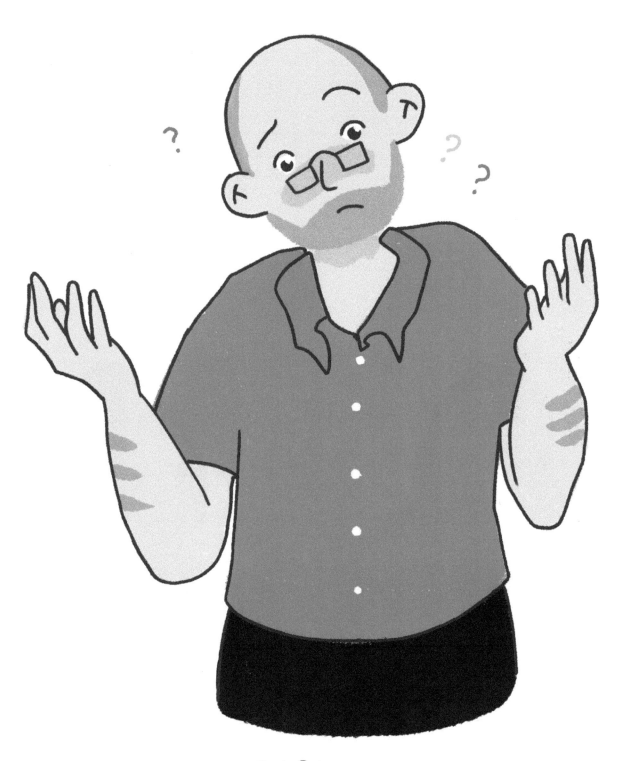

♥ Here is Fiona's Dad, Peter. Typically wondering what all the fuss is about. ♥

Introduction: What's All the Fuss about These Labels Anyway?

By no means do I want to give the impression that New York City made me bisexual, but I was living in New York City when I came to realize that I'm bisexual.

For six years prior I'd been living in Houston, Texas and identified as gay, sometimes using the label lesbian, but I had definitely sworn off men. So much so, I had excited conversations with close friends about the joy of never having to be physically intimate with men again!

When I came out in 2004, being a part of the Houston LGBTQIA+ (although back then we said GLBT) community gave me a sense of belonging and a home where I felt that I could be myself and be loved for who I was. My employment and volunteer work raising money, managing events, and lobbying lawmakers on our issues earned me the community's support and the honor of serving as the 2009 Female Grand Marshal for the Houston LGBTQ+ Pride Parade. I was *that* gay.

For eight years I was out of touch with any unexplored indications of romantic, emotional, and/or sexual attraction towards anyone who wasn't a woman. I'll also add that at this time, I didn't have any close friends who were transgender or nonbinary in my circle, so please forgive me for explaining in such cis-centric, gender-binary terms. As you'll read in this book, I now know that some women have male genitalia, some men have female genitalia, and some people have a combination, but I just wasn't aware back then.

However, I did *love* the company of my gay male friends even more than hanging with women. I used to say that I was a gay man trapped in a woman's body (even though I was attracted to women, so wrap your head around *that* one, lol) and run around the queer bars and clubs with my guys, loving the attention of being the only flirty female in our crew. I also used to jokingly describe myself as a lipstick lesbian fag hag. Ugh, that's a gross word!

But ten months into living in Manhattan, something had begun to shift. I became increasingly aware within my consciousness of being attracted to guys.

My (not so) secret crush on Cory Booker (he/him) eventually forced me to out myself to my lesbian roommate, Marilyn (she/her). The feelings for Cory were so strong that he made it onto my vision board. And over a decade later he's still on there, lol!

Anyway, in 2012 my attraction towards men started feeling apparent in a way I hadn't experienced since 2004. *Darn it,* I thought. *Am I going to have to be physical with men again?* Finally, I came to realize that the only reason I'd been declining a date with a guy was because I'd told myself that I was a lesbian. But if I was really honest with myself, I still had the capacity to be attracted to men.

There was a moment when I freaked out because I didn't want to lose my gay identity. I was scared of being criticized by our community or accused of having just made up being gay in order to be accepted. After all, I'd spent every year as a lesbian defending that label due to the fact that I was previously married to a man. While it wasn't strategic, a lot of work had been done to establish myself internally and externally as a gay woman. Coming to realize that bisexual was a more accurate label meant that I again had to lose an identity that had become such an integral piece of my being. It was sad, scary, and exciting all at the same time. I didn't know anyone else who had come out as bisexual, so I got onto the proverbial horse, took the reins, and decided to ride on out there with my

bi flag flying. And eventually an audacious bee tattoo indelibly marked into my arm.

Once I'd internally satisfied the qualifier of sex and/or gender not necessarily being a barrier to my attraction towards others, I rested on "bisexual" because there's a B in LGBT. Doh! How had I overlooked this all along? If I'd been more knowledgeable about what being bisexual meant back in 2004, maybe I never would've come out as lesbian. Or if I had, maybe I'd have realized that being a lesbian didn't mean being intimate with male anatomy was off the books, because, hello, some women are assigned male at birth and would quite happily like to keep it that way!

Our genitals do not determine our gender, and yet even within our LGBTQIA+ community, we unwittingly get locked into a binary way of thinking. If only the systems of gender norms hadn't been institutionalized along with race and class by oppressive governments, religious doctrine, or colonization. Maybe then we wouldn't know ourselves as an LGBTQIA+ community, but as people within society who are equally recognized and treated under the law regardless of how our gender, our genitals, or our sexual orientation are biologically created.

But here we are, and the way forward is to come out. I chose to announce that I'm bisexual on YouTube™, although my video looks like it was uploaded by a dinosaur compared to the creative and hilarious #Bisexual TikToks® out there today. Who knew that cuffed jeans, vans, an oversized hoodie, a clear iPhone® case, and a whole host of other signs would give "not straight" youth a safe and liberated way to be seen. I'm thrilled for them, even if I haven't mastered their creative social media wizardry. I'm just sitting here sipping my wine with an admiring smile.

Coming out to yourself and others is not a one and done. Over the years, not only have I come to realize that I have the capacity to be romantically, emotionally, and/or sexually attracted to people of different genders, I've become increasingly aware of the social structures that keep some people in power and other people controlled. The strict binary of social norms being imposed upon us is being chipped away, and I know that I have a role in this work.

The award-winning feature documentary I codirected, *TransMilitary*, was described by the *Texas Observer* as, "... one to watch with your anti-LGBT uncle at Thanksgiving, if you dare."[1] This comment nails why I spent over six years of my life advocating for transgender service members through media. While LGBTQIA+ people are a minority in the United States and around the world, they are surrounded by a majority of their family and friends who love them but just don't understand.

Today, I'm embracing my calling as your Auntie Fiona, the bisexual, female version of Mr. Rogers. The person who can help you explain to that anti-LGBT uncle, or even the supportive but confused parent, or *any* friend or

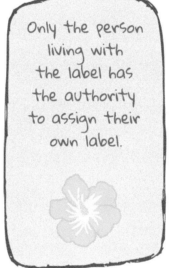

Only the person living with the label has the authority to assign their own label.

family member for that matter, what it means to be LGBTQIA+. Hell, I've heard from some of my LGBTQIA+ friends that even they'd like a few explainers, so I'm writing this book for y'all too. Through my own personal coming-out experiences of feeling straight, then gay, then bisexual, plus my family-you-choose friendships with people who are transgender, nonbinary, or elsewhere on or off the gender and sexuality spectrums, I've learned how to take these concepts and break them down into bare-bones language.

My work is centered around kindness and courage. It's a fact that LGBTQIA+ people face disproportionately higher rates of violence, unemployment, homelessness, poorer physical and mental health outcomes, and so on, and so on. The list of tragedies is horrific. However, while these facts can't be denied, we can't just sink into helplessness and depression. Each of the personal stories behind those statistics includes positive and inspiring people who are doing things to make these situations better.

Studies show that 70 percent of Texans believe that discrimination against LGBT people is wrong,[2] so rather than "fighting hate," I'd like to promote the love that is actually there. In fact, I don't believe all discrimination is based on hate. I believe it's primarily based on a lack of knowledge and levels of fear.

If you call someone a "hater," how do you expect them to respond?

If we want to achieve equity for all people, then I believe we should be empowering people to understand the spectrum of gender and sexuality, rather than mocking those who still see a binary. We should walk our talk and live with love.

My vision for *What Does That LGBTQIA+ Label Mean?* is to break the binary view of gender and sexuality with humor and ease. It's a guide for people who need a very direct, uncomplicated explanation of labels within the LGBTQIA+ community. Although I should make it abundantly clear that this is *not* a guide to help you label someone else. It's a guide so you can understand the label someone gives to themself. Only the person living with the label has the authority to assign their own label.

That being said, you can give this book to anyone old enough to have a very direct conversation about body parts and aspects of humanity. If you're interested in an even franker script, please grab a copy of my first book, *Are Bisexuals Just Greedy?*

But I have a few disclaimers:

♥ This book is not complete. With only 21 chapters, I'm brushing the surface on the most frequently used terms and use *transgender*, *trans*, and *trans** interchangeably, but there are so many more words to explore. Check out the links in the Resources section to find where to do a deeper dive.

♥ This is primarily my perspective, but with a thumbs up from friends who experience the identity I'm describing. I do not claim to be infallible, but I've done my best to read, listen, and understand the research to make sure that I'm not wrong.

♥ While I'm endeavoring to break the binary, I'm ironically sometimes writing in binary terms, as this book is a starting place for people who really know next to nothing. They may understand men being gay, and women being lesbians, but they probably think bisexuals are just greedy. So to all my people who are anywhere on or off the spectrums, I see you. I love you. And I hope this book serves in helping more people in your life appreciate who you are.

I recognize why some people say, "I hate labels," but I believe that they can help. It's not the label that abuses and hurts, it's the speaker. But when spoken with love and positive intention, labels can make us feel visible, embraced, and safe. We can find each other to build community with words to describe our common lived experience. The human brain doesn't like living in an unsolved puzzle, so labels for our gender identity and sexual orientation help our brains create a road map, or even different road maps over time, so we can navigate the world. And of course we need labels to be written into law, healthcare policy, film, television, and all other forms of media to make sure everyone is protected, seen, and heard.

While the terms in this book are not exhaustive, they're a start for people who are curious to know more about being LGBTQIA+. Through the lens of our community, it's my intention that we come to realize that when it comes to gender, genitals, and sexuality, all human beings have them. We just all happen to have been born with different degrees and forms of each.

It's probably best to read the explainers in the order of appearance as I start with the nuts and bolts and build from there. If Uncle Tedd wants to know how transgender women pee in a public restroom, he should probably know the difference between *cisgender* and *transgender* first. You'll notice I saved the extra special answer to "How Can I Keep My Kids Safe from Transgender and Gay People?" for Uncle Tedd last.

That being said, I can imagine one of these topics coming up at your family dinner table and Uncle Tedd wanting to know right then and there if all transgender men want surgery. In which case, you will find much repetition throughout the chapters to help your dear uncle get it while

helping himself to some more gravy, and without you having to start reading the explainers from scratch.

Expect aha moments and giggles from this book. Have it lying on your coffee table, or keep it as part of your library next to the loo. That's British for toilet, y'all. Give it to family members and friends as a gift, or as swag at your next diversity, equity, and inclusion event.

At the end of the day, I encourage you to not take yourself or life too seriously. No matter how grotty the weather is on the ground, the sun is always shining in a brilliant clear sky above the clouds. That same constant love and light exists within us all. Let's make it shine.

Thank you and enjoy!

P.S. Dad, shut your eyes ... Today I feel intimacy in a rich assortment of ways that are not dependent on the anatomy of my partner. Funny how things change.

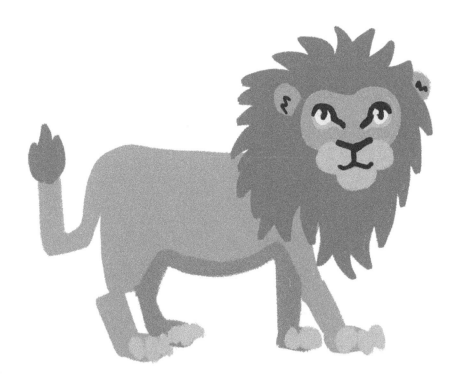

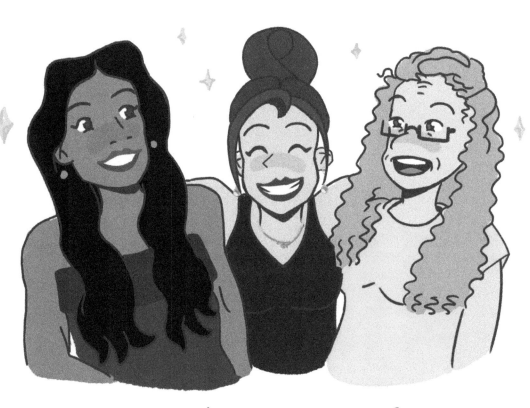

♥ Fiona hugging her Aunty Clare and her friend, Kate. ♥

What's the Difference between "Cisgender" and "Transgender?"

1

My mum, Jane (she/her), was the eldest of four daughters born and raised in London, United Kingdom. Her maiden name was Topp, so when they were in their teens, they were known as "The Four Topps." Get it? As in the Motown group of the 1960s. It's quite amazing to think that an all-Black, male vocal quartet could be compared to four white British girls growing up across the Atlantic. All because of a common name only distinguished by one extra P.

Mum's youngest sister is Clare (she/her). She's my Aunty Clare and also my godmother. Clare has told me many times that I'm the whole reason why she had her first child. When she held me as a baby, she thought I was so cute and felt so much love for me that she had to have one too. She wanted to steal me from my parents but knew that wouldn't fly, so instead she got pregnant at the age of 18 and gave birth to my cousin, Nick (he/him).

Clare sees my Facebook posts from her home in England, so is well aware of my advocacy for LGBTQIA+ people, and especially transgender people like my friend Kate (she/her). Kate is a transgender woman from Honduras who, like me, is an immigrant to the United States. With Kate's willing participation, I've been sharing her story as a way of educating, entertaining, and inspiring people to understand what it means to be transgender. I know Clare is accepting of all people and follows my work closely, but when I asked her if she understood what the word "cisgender" means she wrote back, "Cisgender means moving from male to female. Apparently."

Apparently Clare's Google™ search was not helpful, lol.

So for my amazing godmother Aunty Clare and any of y'all who would love a definition, let's break down the difference between the words "transgender" and "cisgender." Now this is going to be bare-bones and binary, so hold on tight if this is *not* news to you.

Right now, when a baby is born they are assigned a "sex" at birth. Some

1

people are born with female genitalia and some people are born with a male genitalia. And some people, about one in every 100 people born in the United States, are intersex, meaning that they have any variation of male and female sex tissue, chromosomes, and/or hormones.

So currently the baby's genitals are used to proclaim, "It's a boy!" for male genitalia, or "It's a girl!" for female genitalia, and we assign this label for the baby's gender. But the label we assign isn't true for everyone.

This practice is not only scientifically inaccurate, it's actually proving to be quite dangerous given all of the ridiculous antics people are getting up to in gender reveal parties! I mean, people have *died* at freaking gender reveal parties! Just search "died at gender reveal parties" online and you'll see. Plane crashes, exploding pipe bombs, and forest fires have all been to blame. And I'd *love* to know if anyone has actually booed at the puff of pink or blue that is "revealed." I mean, what's going to happen? A disappointed sigh if the unwanted color is the surprise? I get being excited about having a baby, but why on earth are we putting a brand-new human into a box with a bunch of expectations before they've even had a chance to take a breath outside of the womb?!

Just have a bloody baby shower for goodness' sake.

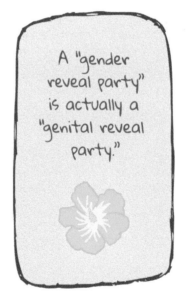

A "gender reveal party" is actually a "genital reveal party."

Because a "gender reveal party" is actually a "genital reveal party." It's saying, "Yay! Our baby has male genitalia!" Or "Yay! Our baby has female genitalia!" And completely overrides the fact that the baby's genitals may be unclear and/or intersex. All we are describing is what the baby's junk looks like, which is kinda personal information to be sharing with the world!

Because *sex* is between the legs, and *gender* is between the ears—i.e. wired into our brains.[1]

Most people grow up feeling that their gender, which is in their heads, is the same as their sex, which is between their legs. So they don't even question it. The label for this is a *cisgender* person. Most people in the world are cisgender. And as Aunty Clare knows from changing my nappies (that's diapers to y'all Americans), I am cisgender.

But some people grow up and come to realize that even though they have female genitalia, their brain knows that they are a boy. Or even though they have male genitalia, their brain knows that they are a girl. The label for this is a *transgender* person.

And transgender people, or anyone who is not cisgender, have to dig deep to realize that it's society that's wrong and then find huge courage to express their true gender to the world. Which is why as an ally to transgender people, I choose to be "out" about being cisgender.

When transgender (also known as "trans") people are expected to label themselves but cisgender (also known as "cis") people are not, we're saying that cisgender is the benchmark for normal and transgender is not normal. In fact, neither is normal; they're just different. Like "The Four Tops" and "The Four Topps." Cisgender just happens to be more typical than transgender, but we have to talk about both in order to create balance in society and not bucket a group of people as outsiders or "others."

So Aunty Clare, and all of y'all my dear friends, Kate is a transgender woman, and I am a cisgender woman. We are both women and have the same gender in our heads; we were just born with different genitals between our legs. And that's very personal, so you can stop thinking about our private parts now, thank you very much!

P.S. I made this Chapter One into an explainer video with Animator EG Smyth (she/they). Check it out, y'all, and share with everyone you know: bitly.com/CisTransExplainer.

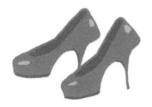

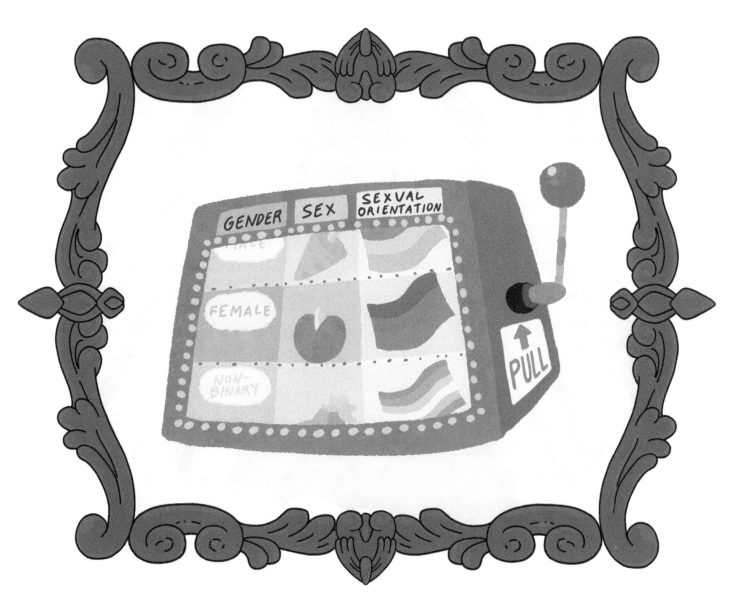

♥ Fiona's imagination of a human slot machine. ♥

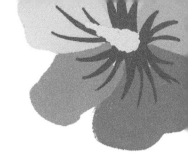

Is Being Transgender the Same as Being Gay?

2

To my LGBTQIA+ family, you've probably heard this question a few times. Still today the word "gay" is used as an umbrella term to dump all of us into one "not straight" bucket. It screams at many of us bisexuals. Look at any mainstream news article reporting on an LGBTQIA+ topic and you'll read "the gay community," but in fact many transgender people are straight!

You see, all humans, including straight people, have three defining parts of their being.

♥ Number one: gender, that's wired in our brains. It's who we know ourselves to be. How we express ourselves to the world. And how the world sees us.

♥ Number two: sex—also known as genitals—lovingly created and visible between our legs. And of course, internally as organs, chromosomes, and hormones that run throughout our entire body.

♥ Number three: sexual orientation. That's invisible to the eye and operates throughout our whole body. It's feelings of romantic, emotional, and/or sexual attraction towards other people.

Each one of these three things exists upon a spectrum.

Some people know that their gender is 100 percent masculine, some people know that they're 100 percent feminine, and others know that their gender feels anywhere in between. Or not at all.

Regarding genitals, some people are born with male genitalia and some people are born with female genitalia. And about one in every 100 people born in the United States are intersex, meaning that they have any variation of male and female sex tissue, chromosomes, and/or hormones. To put it another way, one in 100 people born in the United States have bodies that do not fit into the typical male or female genital and hormone classifications. Really not that surprising when you think about all the other variations of our body parts. Hell, my thighs have always been atypically large compared to my peers.

And when it comes to sexual orientation, some people know that they are straight. Some people know that they are gay or lesbian, and many people identify as bisexual—like me!—meaning that they have the capacity to be attracted to people with the same or a different gender and/or genitals.

To put it *very* basically and bluntly, your gender is who you go to bed as, and your sexual orientation is who you like to go to bed with.

All of these identities are good and valid.

So is being transgender the same as being gay? No. Being transgender means that your gender is different from the label other people gave you when you were born. Being gay means you're attracted to people who have the same or similar gender as you.

Regardless of whether we're straight, gay, lesbian, bisexual, pansexual, cisgender, transgender, or any other identity, just like a three-reel slot machine, we all have a unique combination of gender, genitals, and sexual orientation. But unlike a slot machine, every one of those combinations is a real winner!

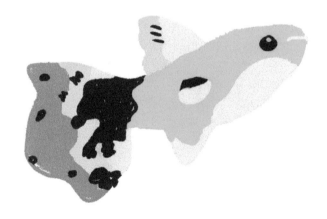

How Do I Know What My Gender Is?

3

This might seem like a silly question, but, in 2013, at the Los Angeles Pride Parade, I was asked, "How do you know that you're a woman?" Today I regret what I wrote.

At that time I said my big hips, small waist, and apparent breasts made me feel like a woman. I tried to dig deeper to find something profound and talked about my feminine strength, compassion for others, kindness for those in need. And finally, stumbling for remarks, I simply wrote, "I just know." And those last three words were actually the greatest truth.

You see, gender is three things:

♥ Number one: who you know yourself to be.

♥ Number two: how you express yourself to the world.

♥ Number three: how the world sees you.

Let's unpack this.

Currently when a baby is born, we examine between their legs to exclaim if they're male, female, or intersex.

This is called "Sex Assigned at Birth" or "SAAB." But all we're describing is what the baby's genitals look like, which as I've said before, is kinda personal information to be sharing with the world. Because sex is between our legs and gender is between our ears, i.e. wired into our brains.

If a baby is born with female genitalia, they are typically "Assigned Female at Birth" or "AFAB."

If a baby is born with male genitalia, they are typically "Assigned Male at Birth" or "AMAB."

Just because I was declared female at my birth, unbeknownst to my parents, they really couldn't know if I was a girl or a boy or another gender until I was old enough to express my gender to the world. Our sense of gender can also be fluid and change over time. Although it's wired into our brains, for some people it's not necessarily fixed at the same spot their whole life.

But throughout my life, I've always felt female. I had a strong knowing of being a girl when I was younger and today of being a woman that I've never even questioned. Since I was AFAB, and I know myself to be a woman, that makes me cisgender.

Let's look at number two, how you express yourself to the world.

Well, I've been influenced by media, fashion, and images of femininity. I made my dad so mad as a teenager wanting to wear short skirts and tight tops, but that's how I was trying to express my growing womanhood to the world.

Expression includes our natural-born mannerisms and attraction to color, sights, scents, and sounds, but is also influenced by what society says is masculine, feminine, and all in between. The magazine makes the bright red lipstick look very pretty to me, but when I wear it, I also just feel more like myself, even when I'm sitting at home alone. And this feeling comes from within my mind, and not from my private parts.

Now, let's move on to number three, how the world sees you.

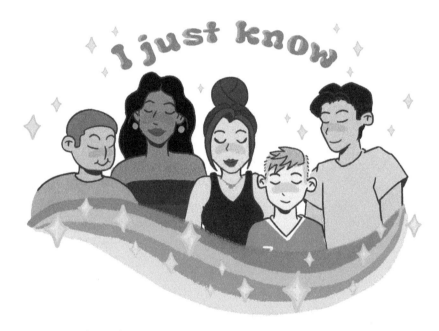

♥ Fiona with Kai, Kate, her nephew Oscar, and illustrator Syd. ♥

Based upon your expression as described in number two, people "read" your gender as male, female, or somewhere else upon the spectrum. People pick up on the cues we give as we conduct ourselves in the world. Society has constructed gender norms, and we label each other according to such.

In fact, it's society that says my big hips, small waist, and apparent breasts

make me a woman. And society that says the way I walk, the way I talk, the clothes I wear, the lipstick I flash, make me a woman. But screw that. I reject what society says is feminine. I'm a woman because "I just know." And *you* are the gender you are because *you* just know. And we should all be able to joyfully and safely express our true gender to the world—wherever that may be on or off the glorious spectrum, in my humble opinion!

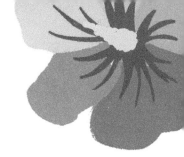

What's the "QIA" in "LGBTQIA"?

4

Actually, if you want to be *even more* inclusive, you should know what "LGBTQIA2S" is!

Lemme help …

L = Lesbian

G = Gay

B = Bisexual

T = Transgender

Q = Queer (can also be Questioning)

I = Intersex

A = Asexual and/or Aromantic (hotly debated if it can also be Ally)

2S = Two-Spirit

This acronym, my friends, is the intersection of gender, genitals, and sexuality.

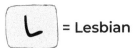 **= Lesbian**

Someone whose gender is female and they have the capacity to be romantically, emotionally, and/or sexually to some degree attracted to people who also have a female gender.

Doesn't matter what their genitals look like.

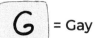 **= Gay**

Someone whose gender is male and they have the capacity to be romantically, emotionally, and/or sexually to some degree attracted to people who also have a male gender.

Doesn't matter what their genitals look like.

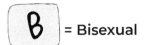 **= Bisexual**

Someone of any gender and they have the capacity to be romantically, emotionally, and/or sexually to some degree attracted to people of the same or a different gender.

Doesn't matter what their genitals look like.

Also note here *Pansexual*, which is like the non-identical twin of bisexual. The definition of pansexual is: Someone of any gender and they have the capacity to be romantically, emotionally, and/or sexually to some degree attracted to people of all genders.

Doesn't matter what their genitals look like.

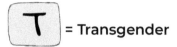 **= Transgender**

Someone whose gender is different from the one other people said it was at their birth. Because dude, gender is something we know and feel on the inside and no one else can define for us.

Btw, *Trans**, as in Trans with an asterisk, is how we reflect the spectrum of gender identities. It's an umbrella term meaning there are countless labels for people who are not cisgender. It's a way of including all those people in one word, which is pretty damn difficult. Our words are not always perfect, but we're doing our best.

Basically, Trans* and Transgender = Not cisgender.

We should also include *nonbinary* people here. Nonbinary people know their gender is not 100 percent male nor 100 percent female. They know their gender is somewhere on the spectrum between those two binary opposites, or completely removed from the gender spectrum altogether.

Some nonbinary people consider themselves transgender and some don't. This is because being nonbinary is a gender identity wired in their brains, whereas sex is visible between their legs. Some nonbinary people *do not* identify with their sex assigned at birth (SAAB) and would say they are transgender. Some nonbinary people *do* partially identify with their sex assigned at birth (SAAB) so say they are not transgender. Nonbinary can be written as "NB" or "Enby," btw.

Doesn't matter what their genitals look like.

 = Queer (can also be Questioning)

Someone who wants to use this word to describe how they feel not straight and/or not cisgender. Not everyone agrees upon this word and it can be painfully insulting to some. Read more about the term queer in Chapter Five.

Doesn't matter what their genitals look like.

The label "Questioning" can be used by someone who knows they're not straight but hasn't found the label that feels right yet (we all need time to figure this stuff out sometimes), so they might say they're questioning this whole gender and sexuality thing.

Doesn't matter what their genitals look like.

 = Intersex

Someone who has any combination of male and female sex tissue, chromosomes, and/or hormones. Yes, that's including their private parts so respect boundaries with your interrogation, please. But btw, know that this untypical variation occurs as frequently as a person being born with red hair. You've probably met someone who is intersex.

Doesn't matter what their genitals look like.

= Asexual and/or Aromantic (hotly debated on if it can also be Ally)

Asexual is someone who experiences between very little to zero sexual attraction.

Doesn't matter what their genitals look like.

Aromantic is someone who experiences between very little to zero romantic attraction.

Doesn't matter what their genitals look like.

Ally. All right, this is hotly debated but I'm gonna go there.

By definition, an ally is someone who does not identify as LGBTQIA+ but takes action in heart, mind, body, and/or soul to support those who do. There's a spectrum of allies too.

The disagreement over the A representing "ally" revolves around whether the word has a place within an acronym that already fails to include every single one of our identities.

Some people do not believe that cisgender, heterosexual people should take up space in our growing yet still limited acronym. Asexual and aromantic people, like many within our community, have not been visibly seen and heard, so adding non-queer people to our acronym dilutes their inclusion, again.

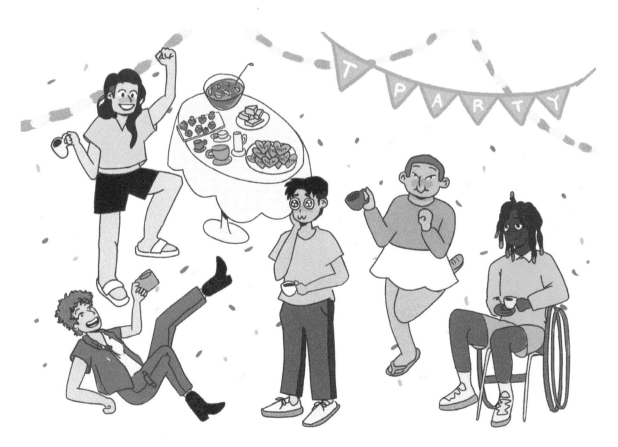

♥ Syd centered in their "T-Party" with their partner and friends. ♥

Personally, I question if anyone on this planet is 100 percent cisgender and heterosexual, especially as we uncover attraction being the capacity to be romantically, emotionally, and/or sexually *to some degree* attracted to people. We all belong on or off the gender, genital, and sexuality spectrums, just some of us have been marginalized and treated like shit for a long time. But I'll save that discourse for another book.

The selling factor for me in not including ally here is the difference between action and identity. Being an ally is something you choose to do with action. Being LGBTQIA2S (or not cisgender and heterosexual) is an identity. And in this case we're talking about identity. In other cases I believe it's important to welcome allies at our inclusion table too. Great things happen when we work together, so know I love and appreciate all of y'all.

Doesn't matter what their genitals look like.

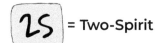 **= Two-Spirit**

A word representing a number of other labels specifically used by indigenous people for someone who has any combination of male and female genders. Look forward to the "Is Being Nonbinary Just Cool These Days?" chapter for more on being Two-Spirit.

Doesn't matter what their genitals look like.

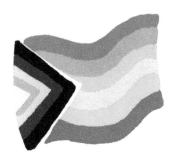

What Does the Word "Queer" Mean?

5

The word queer can mean different things to different people, but some are wondering what it represents in the LGBTQIA+ acronym, so I'll do my best to explain how different humans use the word queer.

First, let's establish what we mean when we say LGBT, or lesbian, gay, bisexual, and transgender. In some ways I wish we could just say that this is everyone who's not straight, but that would be a disservice to all of the beautiful identities existing upon our spectrums. And some transgender people are straight.

If we take the first three letters, we're reflecting sexual orientation. I'm actually going to add S in this explanation. Yup! S for straight, because straight people are included here too, and you'll see why in a bit.

So, straight people, as we know by now, are people who have the capacity to experience sexual, romantic, and/or love feelings towards someone of a different gender.

Side note: it's commonly said of the "opposite" gender, but we should really do away with that as it implies there are only two genders opposing one another, and biologists now know that there are actually an uncountable number of genders.

Lesbian and gay people have the capacity to experience sexual, romantic, and/or love feelings towards someone of the same or similar gender.

And bisexual people—like me!—have the capacity to experience sexual, romantic, and/or love feelings towards someone of the same gender and/or a different gender.

So that's basically sexual orientation. *Very* basically.

Then we get to the fourth letter in the acronym, the T, representing gender identity.

T stands for transgender. A transgender person is someone whose gender is different from the one people assumed it was going to be based upon their genitals when they were born. If we were to be more balanced, we'd actually include C for cisgender here. A cisgender person is someone whose gender is not different from the one people assumed it was going to be based upon their genitals when they were born. Most people in the world are cisgender.

It kind of irks me that when we talk about transgender people, we are forced to bring up their genitals, because that is really rather personal information to be sharing with the world. So to be fair, I think it's only right that cisgender people's junk has to be mentioned here too.

Plus, both cisgender and transgender people can be any sexual orientation, such as those mentioned above like straight, lesbian, gay, bisexual, pansexual, etc.

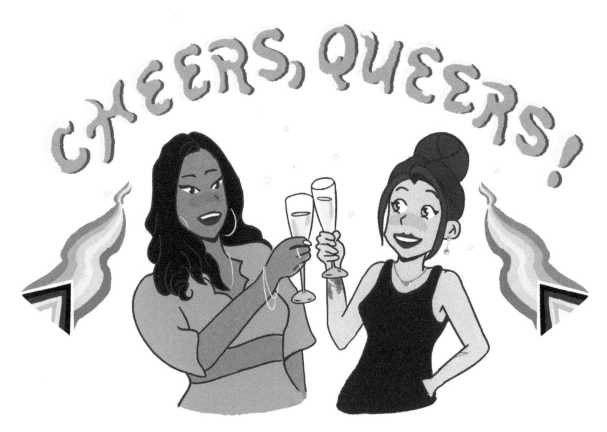

♥ Laila and Fiona clinking flutes as they love to do! ♥

Furthermore, like trans* people, cis people can also identify and express themselves as strictly male, female, or anywhere between, on or off, the gender spectrum. You see, both trans* and cis people can have a binary gender identity or a nonbinary gender identity. Personally, I think cis and trans* humans have a lot more in common than we first think.

But let's move on. Having just established we have a sexual orientation umbrella and a gender identity umbrella, let's consider the word *queer*.

Queer can be used to describe both gender and/or sexual orientation identities that do not fit in a straight and/or cisgender box.

However, it's very important to note that not everyone feels the same way about the word, especially as it has been historically—and still is—used as hate speech and violence against the LGBTQIA+ community. The word can be very painful for some people to hear, but at the same time many others have widely reclaimed and empowered the term and find it very useful to represent the fluidity and complexity of our identities.

For example, I am a cisgender, mostly-femme-gender-expressing, bisexual woman but I sometimes *love* using queer to describe myself as it tells the world I am not who you think I am. I may look typical on the outside, but on the inside I feel like a gender-bending unicorn dressed up as a pirate wench!

And the delish thing about the word is that it means whatever you want it to mean when it comes to blowing up the binary of the gender and sexuality boxes, we *all*—yes, straight, cisgender people included—have been forced to live in for way too long.

With that, I have just one more thing to say: cheers, queers!

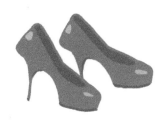

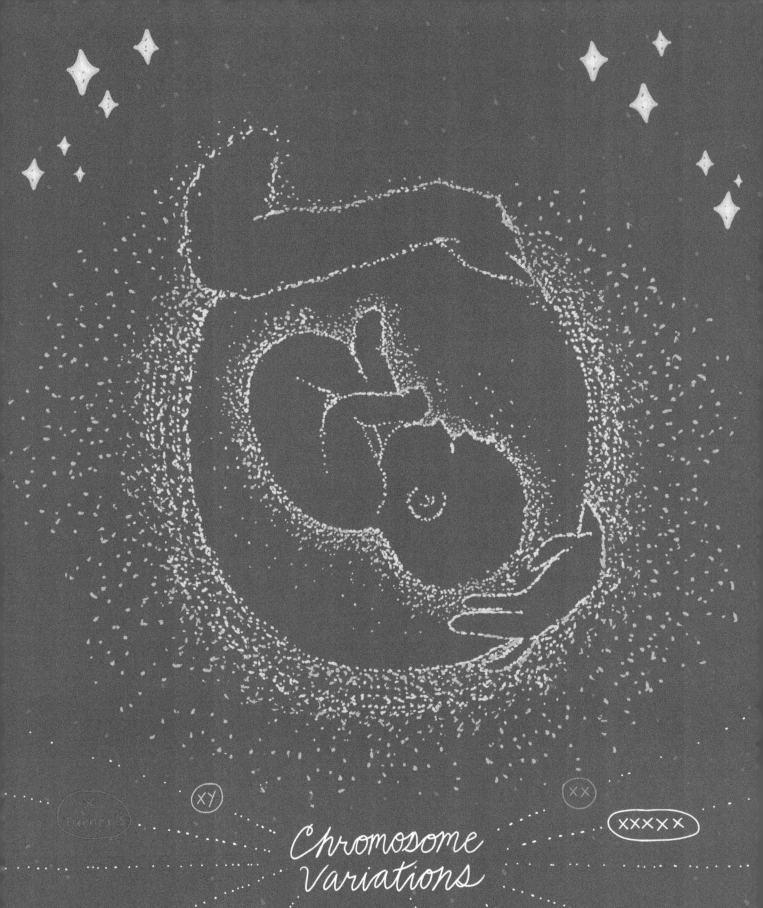

Chromosome
Variations

X
Turner's

XY

XX

XXXXX

XXX
Triple X

XYY
Jacobs
syndrome

XXYY,XXYY
Klinefelter

XXXY,XXXXY
Klinefelter

What Does It Mean to Be Intersex?

6

The miracle that is our junk is formed when we're growing in the womb. It takes a biological, chemical combination to form chromosomes, genitals, and reproductive tissue to determine if we're labeled male with male genitalia or female with female genitalia at our birth.

However, bodies come in so many different shapes, sizes, and colors. From our heads and shoulders to our knees and toes, not one human being has an identical feature to any other human.

We use our bodies in different ways too. Some of us are left-handed, some of us are right-handed, and some people are ambidextrous—meaning they can use both.

Butts are different, boobs are different, and yes, genitals are different too. In fact, the individual differences between anatomy labeled "male" and anatomy labeled "female" are far greater than those genitals that cannot be labeled as either.[1]

That's right. While no male genitalia are identical and no female vaginas are identical, there also exists a spectrum of penises and vaginas in between. Up to 1.7 percent of the world's population[2]—again, about the same number of people who are born with red hair[3]—don't neatly fit into a male or a female category, so they are labeled as "intersex," meaning that they have any variation of male and female sex tissue, chromosomes, and/or hormones. This is not a disorder. This is a *variation*.

Not all intersex people are identical either. Some people may have female chromosomes but male-appearing genitalia. Or male chromosomes but female-appearing genitalia. Some people are born with ovaries and testicles. Some people have a mosaic of XX and XY chromosomes. And some people have a combination undetectable at birth, so they don't even realize they're intersex until puberty. In fact, sex anatomy development can be labeled in over 40 medical terms.[4] Not two.

Because we typically keep our clothes on in public, we simply aren't aware of this sensational spectrum that exists between our legs. We can't tell if the people around us have been labeled male, female, or intersex by judging their expression of gender.

And quite frankly, it's none of our freaking business.

The person most concerned about someone else's genitals should be that someone else—and their chosen and trustworthy health care professional to make sure that they remain in tip top shape!

Additionally, the shape of our genitals doesn't always predict the gender we feel in our brains. In the same way your hands don't dictate if you use your left or your right to write, your genitals don't dictate what kind of gendered clothes you want to wear. Nor the type of person you're attracted to, for that matter! Both gender and sexual orientation are wired in your brain, whereas your sex is cells, chromosomes, and hormones throughout your body.

Unfortunately, even healthcare professionals are taking their time

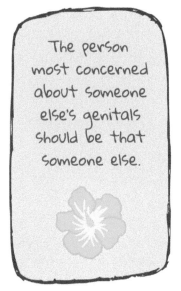

The person most concerned about someone else's genitals should be that someone else.

to move us out of this binary world. For too long, babies and children have had their genitals mutilated because they didn't look like male genitalia or female genitalia the medical professional expected. It's ironic that transgender people are often denied the surgery they need to align their gender and their genitals, while at the same time, intersex children are being sculpted and molded without their consent to make their parts look how society thinks they should be!

So, before we assume that male genitalia makes you a man and female genitalia makes you a woman, regardless of what your private parts look like, let's remember that the beautiful existence of intersex people illustrates that your unique junk is who you are privately, physically designed to be, and your gender is how you publicly express yourself to the world.

Got it? Fantastic!

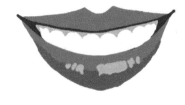

What Do You Mean Some People Don't Want to Have Sexual Relations?

7

It's funny to me that sex is hyped up in so many ways in our culture, and used to sell clothes, shoes, perfume, cars, vacuum cleaners ... and yet we rarely have a safe space to frankly discuss sex as a matter of fact.

If it wasn't for my mother coming home with a picture book one day to teach me how babies were made, and how to make sure babies were *not* made, I would've relied upon our poor high school biology teacher for my sex education. Imagine, one week he's dissecting the anatomy of a rat, and the next he's drawing male genitalia on the chalkboard with 32 giggling 16-year-old girls looking on.

But even though it's a taboo subject to discuss and we're taught in the most sterilized of fashions, it's assumed that everyone is doing it and everyone is loving it. Imagine if we treated sex the same way we approach driving cars, but without the test of course! We're all attracted to—or don't care about—different makes, models, and experiences. Having some lessons certainly helps. Some of us start earlier

than others, and we may, or may not, retire as we age. My dad, who's a retired doctor, told me that he recalls prescribing Viagra® to one of his 90-year-old patients on a fairly regular basis. Wowzers.

However, as with driving, not everyone has the same desire to do it. People who experience little to no attraction towards driving cars identify as non-drivers. People who experience little to no sexual attraction towards other people identify as asexual.

For those of us who are not asexual, to get as close as we can to understanding what it means to be asexual, let's forget about dating, romance, and what we see in the movies for a few hot minutes and instead dive into the human brain to look at the device that is ATTRACTION. We all have one, including straight people.

Imagine inside of your brain there's an ATTRACTION device shaped like a rectangular box. Take the lid off this device, and inside we see three sliding markers that can move along, and even off, their own unique scale thingy. Let's call these scales and markers "spectrums."

Each of these spectrums has a different label.

♥ One is called LOVE.

♥ One is called ROMANCE.

♥ One is called SEX. (As in the behavior, not the genitals in this instance).

The markers are adjustable and can move over time, but when the spectrums are set together, they determine what *attraction* label(s) society will give us. When those attraction labels are compared to our gender, then *they* determine what

sexual orientation label(s) society will give us.

But let's stay focused on just attraction right now.

Each spectrum has the capacity to rest at a different spot, or even leave the spectrum entirely. Some people have a very common combination, some people have a very unique combination, and some people are somewhere in between. But every single one of these combinations is beautiful and magnificent in its existence. This is not a test where anyone can fail, but simply a matter of how we were each designed uniquely by our maker.

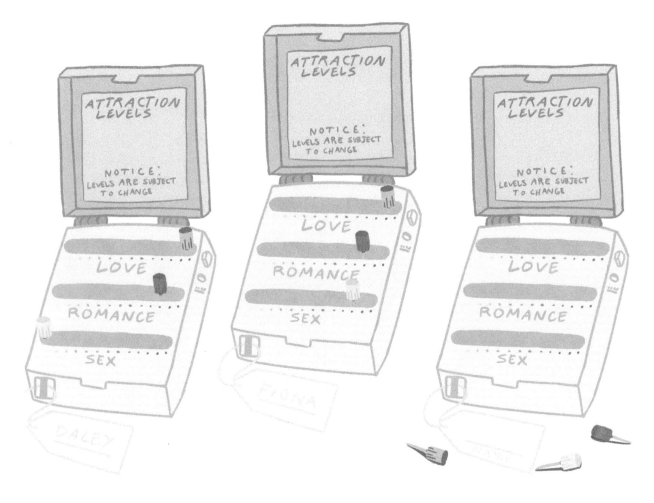

♥ Where would you put your pins within your attraction device? ♥

Let's do a side-by-side comparison of how two people's spectrums can be different, leading to a different sexual *attraction* label. To keep this <ahem> straightforward, I'll use myself and my asexual friend Daley (she/her) as an example. But remember, we're just a sample of two and there are thousands of other possible combinations that exist.

Daley and my LOVE spectrums are both set high meaning we both experience lots of feelings of love. And this could be for anyone … friends, family, significant others, even our pets. But keeping it in the human relationship love category, I'm a big lover. I fall in love with people I date very easily and often say, "I love you" first and early. I can't help it, it just bursts out of me. And Daley says she feels her love spectrum is super-high too, and she loves her husband very deeply indeed.

Now let's look at ROMANCE. This is also set high on both my and Daley's spectrums for both giving and receiving. Although as a side note, I'm aware that I'm influenced by what society says is romantic and much of romance is a social construct, but I digress. Both Daley and I feel new relationship energy heavily. I've become aware of my primary love languages being quality time and words of affirmation, which I want anyone dating me to know pretty quickly! I'd rather receive a sweet hand-written note than a dozen red roses. If my partner texts me a song with loving lyrics, then my heart leaps out of my chest. Daley loves all of these things too, and cuddles by the fireplace, candlelit dinners, and holding hands like love birds with her hubby.

Finally let's turn to the SEX spectrum. Just like the previous LOVE and ROMANCE spectrums, each of us humans has a different capacity for desire to have SEX.

> People who experience little to no sexual attraction towards other people identify as asexual.

The label for people who *do* experience sexual attraction is allosexual. It's assumed that most people in the world are allosexual. Romantic movies and TV shows typically lump love, romance, and sex into the same category, assuming that everyone wants it all. But that's not true for everybody.

People somewhere in the middle can be labelled as *demisexual* or *graysexual*. Demisexual people need to have an emotional bond with someone for the sexual attraction to turn on. Graysexual people sometimes experience sexual attraction, and it might be only within specific situations.

People who experience very little to no sexual attraction are called asexual. Some asexual people do still have consensual sex with the person (or people) that they choose to be with because they feel it's an important part of their relationship. Furthermore, just like allosexual people, asexual people can also be sex workers, because after all, it's a job. We can all do things we're not biologically motivated to do if we put our mind to it. Like me making myself run three miles most mornings so I can eat Pringles® and drink wine.

My SEX spectrum is somewhere between allosexual and demisexual. I love to get it on, and get on it, but I *really* want to do it with the person I have an emotional connection with. Because emotional connection often happens for me as easily as striking a match, it doesn't take long!

Daley, however, would say her SEX spectrum is asexual as she does not experience sexual attraction towards other people. She *is* attracted to people, but it's a physical ache in her chest and not a physical ache in her genitals. This feeling in her chest drives her to want intimacy like holding hands, kissing, and being close with people she's attracted to, it just doesn't drive her to sex. But don't forget, just

> People of any sexual orientation can be allosexual or asexual, or anywhere else on the spectrum of sexual drive.

because she's asexual, like me she still experiences LOVE and ROMANCE attraction towards other people. Each of the three spectrums are independent of each other.

People of any sexual orientation can be allosexual or asexual, or anywhere else on the spectrum of sexual drive. So anyone can be asexual and straight, or asexual and gay, or asexual and lesbian, or asexual and bisexual, or any other orientation because an ATTRACTION box exists in the brains of all people. See how much we all have in common!

Phew, my darling friends. Is this puzzle solved for y'all!?

Essentially, no matter how we're wired, whether we're asexual or not, we're all awesome. We just happen to have our spectrums set at different places within the attraction devices inside our heads.

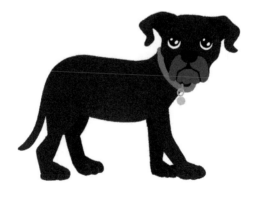

Do Transgender Men Actually Exist?

8

I'm friends with quite a few and dated a couple, so I can confidently assure you that transgender men definitely exist. And in some ways, they're really not that much different from the cisgender men I know and have dated either.

A transgender man is someone who was born with female genitalia or could have been labeled intersex if their genitals didn't neatly fit into one of the two very limited options on a certificate of birth. Typically, society assumes that they are a girl because they have female genitalia, but as they grow up they realize that their gender, which is actually programmed in their brain and not between their legs (doh!), is male. This makes them a transgender man.

Today, transgender women are much more visible in media as actresses and celebrities than transgender men. And these women are also being more severely attacked through societal structures and outright violence, especially those women who are not white. While killings of trans* and nonbinary people are massively underreported, the numbers are still horrific in comparison to their population, and over 90 percent of those we can count are Black and/or Latina women.[1] However, transgender men probably exist in about equal numbers within society;[2] we just don't as frequently recognize them as trans when we're casually passing by.

One of the biggest reasons for this is physical changes. When someone chooses to medically transition with life-saving hormone therapy, if they have already gone through puberty, their body's ability to change is affected by the level of testosterone and/or estrogen that they naturally produce. Changes in the body as a teen due to testosterone are much harder to change again than those produced by estrogen.

Let's break down what I mean here, but I'll start by stating a fact: no irreversible surgical intervention ever happens to non-intersex transgender children before or during puberty.[3] Ever.

When kids hit puberty, it can become extremely distressing for a transgender boy if they start developing breasts and/or start a period due to estrogen hormone changes. Society says men don't have boobs or periods, so a guy growing a pair and/or needing tampons can make someone feel really grossed out. Actually, that's just putting it mildly.

Trigger warning: Studies report over half of transgender and nonbinary youth seriously consider suicide[4] ... all because the adults in the room don't understand that gender and biological sex are different and fail to support our young people.

If you are a young person considering suicide, please call the TrevorLifeline at 1-866-488-7386 or text "START" to 678-678 right now.

If you are over twenty-five years old and considering suicide, please call the National Suicide Prevention Lifeline at 1-800-273-8255 or text 988 right now.

Everyone else, let's focus on the positive ways of embracing transmasculinity.

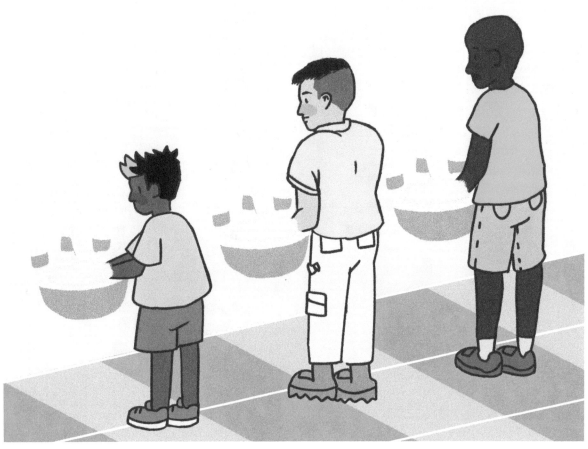

♥ Technical Sergeant Logan Ireland, a member of the Department of the Air Force Office of Special Investigations (OSI), wisely washes his hands. ♥

One of the ways transgender men, nonbinary, and transmasculine people can make their chest feel more comfortable and masculine is to start "binding." There are a number of safe ways they can do this using binders, which are unique garments specifically designed to shape their chest like a masculine torso. Imagine a compression tank top. Easily found on the internet if you want a picture.

As for periods, even though sanitary towel and tampon dispensers are typically only in the women's restroom, let's remember that some men have periods too. As a side note, thankfully diaper-changing stations are becoming more common in the men's facilities, acknowledging that some men do also change diapers. Some men even change the diapers of the beloved baby they gave birth to. Fancy that!

But when it comes to that potentially dreaded time of the month, there's also a very easy, safe, and reversible solution for teens who are psychologically traumatized by their ovulation. Puberty blockers. This life-saving medicine was actually stumbled upon in some unrelated research, and then first used as a "pause button" for children who were beginning puberty as early as preschool.[5] Yes, many human bodies are born on their own unique timeline. This pause button is proven to be completely safe and if stopped at any time, puberty resumes from where it left off.

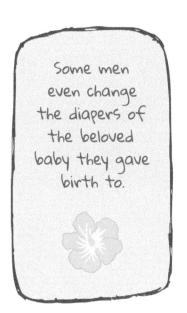

Some men even change the diapers of the beloved baby they gave birth to.

For most young boys who do start blockers, it gives them a chance to think deeper before it's too late to prevent a female form from developing within their skin. And of course, the same applies to young girls who would be traumatized from growing body hair and a larger penis. This time is **critical** in preventing bullying, self-harm, and even suicide.[6]

After thinking about it carefully during this pause on puberty, and also privately consulting with their medical professional like any other person would do about a serious condition, most teens later decide to accept a prescription of gender-affirming hormones.[7] For trans men and masculine-centered individuals, this means that they can start taking testosterone to help their bodies reach a hormonal level that appropriately matches their gender. And for trans women and feminine-centered individuals, they can take estrogen to help their bodies reach a hormonal level that appropriately matches their gender. Kinda like how some people need to take insulin to help their bodies reach a sugar level that appropriately matches their internal organs.

When they reach the right balance of testosterone in their body—something that is figured out privately with their healthcare professional and none of our freaking business—feelings of self-harm typically decrease and trans men start to develop all the typical characteristics we label as masculine. Like facial hair—actually, hair everywhere—a deeper voice, broad shoulders, and muscles. Big ones if they work out like some of those cisgender guys in the gym. But just like the cis guys, they have to work out! The T just aligns their internal sense of gender, making them feel happier inside their body but not necessarily building big muscles. It's the bench presses, protein shakes, and determination that produce the guns!

After several months to a year, trans* guys start to walk the world and people see them as male. They easily "blend in." This can be called "passing" and the ability to blend in is called by some "passing privilege." However, there is debate on the use of these labels given that they reinforce society's acceptance of the gender binary. The concept of it being a privilege to not get attacked because of how you look is a very sad reflection of humanity to me.

For trans women who've already experienced the effects of testosterone, it's a little more challenging to transition their bodies into what society says is feminine, so we see trans women more visibly in the world.

But all along since birth, trans women have been women, and trans men have been men. They simply needed medical care to help their bodies align with their gender. Similar to the millions of cisgender people who take hormone therapies to help with their physical, emotional, and sexual selves, too.

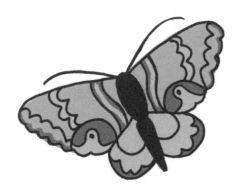

Is Being Nonbinary Just Cool These Days?

9

Last week, a guy in his 20s texted me, "What is binary and nonbinary?"

I replied:

"Binary means only two options. In gender, binary is 100 percent "male" or 100 percent "female." Nonbinary is someone who is not 100 percent male or female. They're somewhere in between."

He replied:

"So how would you address a nonbinary person? Do they not like to be called he or she?"

I replied:

"Typically no. Nonbinary people usually want to be called they/them. There are other pronouns too, but they/them is usual."

He replied:

"What other pronouns would you call them?"

I replied:

"Pronouns such as xe, ze, sie, co, and ey are sometimes used as well. But I have not learned them all."

We then started texting about the weather.

The beautiful illustrations in this book are created by my friend, Syd (they/them). Syd is nonbinary and shared with me that some people, regardless of their body parts, feel that they have no gender at all, or that their gender is fluid. People who feel this way often identify as gender nonconforming, nonbinary, agender, genderqueer, or genderfluid, or any other label that feels right to them. The Williams Institute recently found that "a greater percentage of nonbinary LGBTQ adults are cisgender rather than transgender."[1]

Essentially, human beings come in all different shapes, sizes, pronouns, and identities. And each person is worthy and valuable.

It's fascinating that this is being discussed like it's a new fad, because being nonbinary has always been cool all over the world! In fact hundreds of years ago, it was so chill that nonbinary was just another accepted identity.

There wasn't even an expectation of gender to conform to. But tragically, white colonists like my forebears attempted to beat these people out of existence.

I've had the mind-opening experience of living and working in a village with Mande tribal people in Bangladesh, whose social structure was matriarchal,[2] meaning that women had the power that we see in a patriarchal society— they owned the land, their husbands took their last names when they married, and their daughters inherited their property upon their death. They flipped the binary.

In India I interviewed and danced with Hijra, trans women recognized as having a third gender and deeply respected for their place in society.[3] Their existence, which has been documented for over 4,000 years, writes nonbinary gender firmly into history.

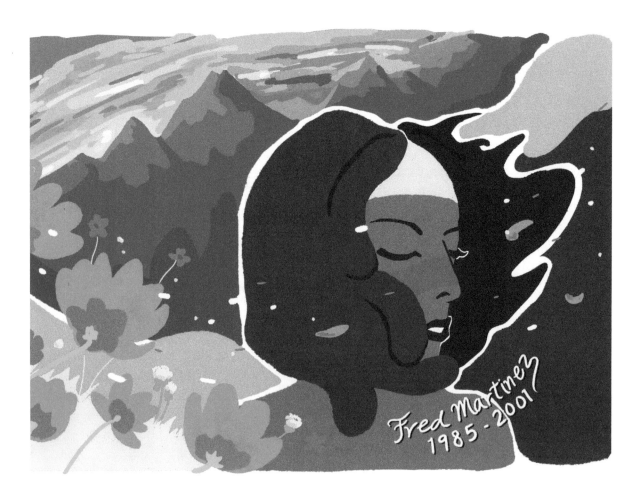

Fred Martinez
1985 - 2001

Across the world, indigenous people, aka the OG peoples of the planet, did not have two strict gender boxes into which every person must fit. Trans* people were documented thousands of years before Jesus was documented.[4]

While women and men were known for their unique contributions to society, they were not confined by the social structures that were later imposed upon them. And the gray area of gender was acknowledged and included.

Now I don't want to paint too rosy a picture as we know horrific acts of violence happened too. However, essentially, before colonization, cultures around the world already had a concept of gender and biological sex as being nonbinary. They were doing just fine, thank you very much. People were liberated to express their internal sense of self as they wished. Intersex people were not forced into nonconsensual surgery. And Two-Spirit individuals were put on a pedestal for their binary-breaking superpowers.

Now I've gotta say some more here, because Two-Spirit people illustrate how native people had this whole gender and sexuality thing down before my ancestors came along and royally ruined it all with their silly rules saying men do this and women do that.

Back in the day (like hundreds of years ago), Two-Spirit individuals were held in very high esteem, worshipped even, as having magical connections to spirituality across the Universe. Some would say they had a direct line to God. They brought people together in love, they cured illness, they kicked effing ass in wars. And they brought peace.

The word Two-Spirit was adopted in 1990 to be helpful in representing people of many different genders with different names. As non-native people had a hard time pronouncing and understanding all the concepts, the good people at the "Third Annual Native American Gay and Lesbian Gathering" made it easy on us and determined the term "Two-Spirit."[5]

Being a white European woman living in this century in the United States, I can't take back what my people did, but I can help expose history. Non-native people such as the colonists that "discovered" the Americas imposed not only violence and genocide against indigenous people who'd already been living on this land for centuries, and then stole African people from their homes and made them work as slaves, but they also forced strict rules within two buckets for gender—male and female—and one bucket for sexuality; straight.

Now we know better. Those colonists had it all wrong. It's time to open the curtain and realize that there's actually a whole stage full of people of different races, ethnicities, and cultures, with a natural spectrum of gender, genitals, and sexuality who've been here all along. Love thy neighbor, my friends. There's room on this stage for us all. And decolonize gender, genitals, and sexuality.

Remember, in America, native people had been living on the land for thousands of years and are only called "Indians" because Columbus had his bearings all wrong and thought he'd ended up in India![6] Some Native nations not only recognized Two-Spirit individuals but had words for five or more genders.

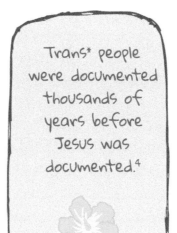

Trans* people were documented thousands of years before Jesus was documented.[4]

It was the colonists who swooped in hundreds of years ago with their "women do this" and "men to that" attitude that destroyed it all!

So next time someone comes out as gender nonbinary or nonconforming, give them kudos for being "woke," and celebrate their authenticity and courage for refusing to be controlled by a bunch of colonists dating back to the 15th century!

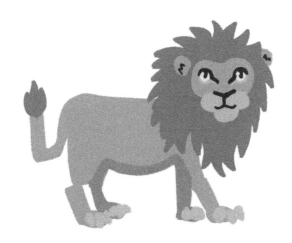

Are Drag Queens Transgender?

10

At WorldPride 2019 in New York City, I made a new friend, Dixie Krystals (she/her). Dixie named herself after the little pink sugar packets from back in the 1950s. Seeing as I grew up in the United Kingdom in the 1980s, I had absolutely no idea what she was talking about, but that didn't matter. They sounded whimsical and we moved on.

Dixie's from Denver and has been doing drag for 21 years. Her self-described brand is "campy queen," and as you can tell from Syd's illustration, she's quite ... well ... subtle, lol. Just kidding! Come on, she's dressed like a freaking loofah and at my height of five foot one, she would make a fantastic personal full-body shower sponge. I wouldn't even have to use my hands!

After experimenting with her skirt for size, I asked Dixie what labels she gives herself. "Gay," she said.

I inquired further, "Just gay, gay, gay?"

Dixie confirmed, "Gay, gay, gay, gay all the way. Yes. Absolutely."

Because I have to get to the bottom of everything, no pun intended, I asked for clarification, "A gay man?"

Dixie confirmed, "Gay man, yes."

And to take this completely into TMI, this gay man also happens to be born with male genitalia, so Dixie is a cisgender—not a transgender—gay man.

If at this point you're confused, let's untangle the threads of gender, genitals, and sexual orientation.

Let me tell you about John (he/him). He grew up in the small town of Curwensville, Pennsylvania. He was assigned male at birth because he was born with male genitalia, which is really just circumstantial and very private information! As John developed, he never questioned his gender, which is wired in his brain. He always knew he was a boy, dressed as a boy, and people saw him as a boy. Boy, boy, boy, boy. Born with both male genitalia and a brain that society says is male, it means he's cisgender.

But John also found that he was attracted to males. When he started dating, he only dated people of the same gender. Other men. So his sexual orientation is gay.

So why on earth did John (he/him), a gay man, decide to become Dixie (she/her) and dress like a woman? Well to start with, John, like many actors, always dreamed of having their name in lights. They were trained in musical theatre and worked for various entertainment companies and regional playhouses. And they just love the feeling of pretending to be a woman. But that's the difference. Drag queens are giving the illusion of being a woman. Transgender women are women.

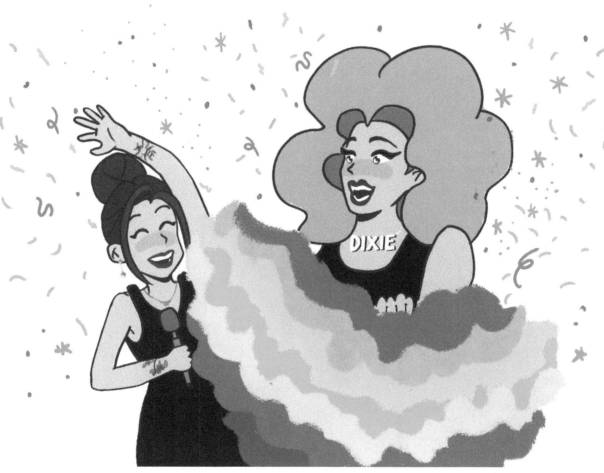

♥ Fiona and Dixie Krystals at WorldPride 2019 in New York City. ♥

Men have actually been dressing up to perform as women for hundreds of years. Originally because women weren't allowed to be actors, which is sexist and sucks. So men played the women's roles, and today some of them still revel in the entertainment and artistic performance of it all.

But John, whose performance name is Dixie Krystals, also uses Dixie's voice to inspire younger generations by hosting drag queen story time in public libraries for kids and their parents. She reads children's books about inclusion and acceptance, educating on the beautiful diversity of families within the neighborhood. She wants to proudly show that there are many sides to someone who's six foot four, wearing a dress, wig, and heels. She gives hope to young people that we're creating a world where they can be true to themselves.

However at the end of the day, when Dixie steps off her stage, she's back to happily being John, a gay dude. Just like the World Wrestling Entertainment's *The Undertaker* is back to being Mark Calaway when he steps out of the ring, a drag queen takes off their makeup to be themselves.

It's not the same for transgender women.

Like cisgender women, trans women are born with a gender wired in their brains that tells them that they are a

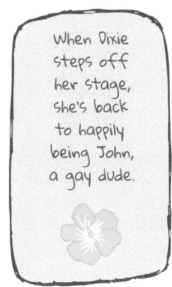

When Dixie steps off her stage, she's back to happily being John, a gay dude.

woman. That means unless they had the fortune of transitioning at a young age, the performance they've had to work at the hardest is that of being a man.

However, remember that John's story is just one example of being a drag queen. As with everything in life, there's not just one or two types of people who enjoy performing in drag. People of all gender identities including masculine, nonbinary, feminine, and the some 61 other known gender labels;[1] and all sexual orientations like gay, straight, lesbian, bisexual, pansexual, etc. etc. etc.; and all sexes-assigned-at-birth (SAAB) such as cisgender, transgender, intersex; could enjoy performing drag. Basically, *any* human being. The key to remember is that drag is a performance and not necessarily a person's identity in real life.

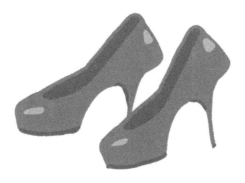

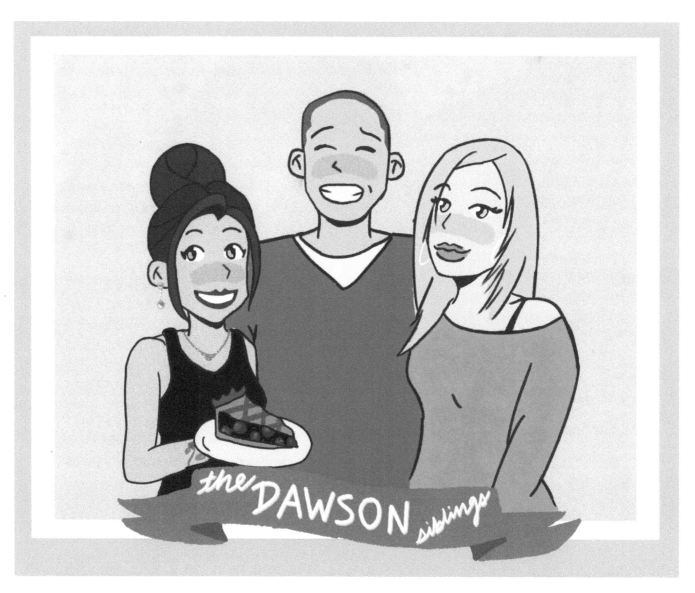

♥ Fiona with her younger siblings Joey and Rob. ♥

Are Bisexuals Just Greedy?

11

When I was a teenager, my dad said to me, "I can understand men being gay and I can understand women being lesbians, but I think bisexuals are just greedy." So Dad, with lots of love from your bisexual daughter, this bare-bones and binary explainer is just for you.

When I was born, my parents saw me as their beautiful baby girl. I was assigned female at birth, was put into dresses, and grew up expressing feminine traits. Well, for the most part! All told, like most people in the world, I've always felt that my sex assigned at birth and my gender matched. Therefore, I am a cisgender woman.

But being a cisgender woman does nothing to predict my sexual orientation. Our sexuality is another matter entirely. You see, all human beings have three different components to our sexual orientation:

💜 Number one: our ATTRACTION.

Attraction is our capacity for love, romance, and/or sexual feelings determined by our genes and hormones, i.e. wired into our brains. (Definitely check out Chapter Seven to unpack ATTRACTION).

Not everyone has the same degrees of attraction towards other people.

Some people do experience attraction, some people don't experience attraction, and everyone else falls somewhere in between.

💜 Number two: our IDENTITY.

This is the sexual orientation label we give to ourselves based on who we're attracted to when compared to our own gender. (For a more detailed explanation, check out Chapter Four).

Most people are straight, meaning that they have the capacity to be attracted to someone of a different gender.

Some people are gay or lesbian, meaning that they have the capacity to be attracted to someone of the same gender.

And people like me are bisexual, meaning that we have the capacity to be attracted to someone of a different or the same gender, which is really quite common. In fact, studies show that within the lesbian, gay, and bisexual (LGB) community, over half of those people identify as bisexual.[1]

Yes, you read that correctly, most LGB people identify as bisexual. But we're assumed to be either gay or straight depending on the gender expression of the person we're dating. We bi+ people are on the receiving end of a whole array of awful stigma and discrimination, especially from our lesbian and gay counterparts. My identity was even put down by a gay woman I was dating when she said something so explicit and rude I can't even put it in this version of my book! (Check out my first version, *Are Bisexuals Just Greedy?* if you really want to know. Or just message me.)

Anyway, that leads me on to behavior.

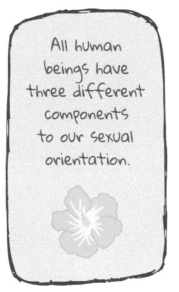

All human beings have three different components to our sexual orientation.

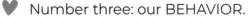 Number three: our BEHAVIOR.

Behavior is how we act upon our attraction and identity. Regardless of sexual orientation, most people in the world, myself included, are not attracted to *everyone* they meet and want to be in a relationship with just one person. Some people want to consensually, ethically, and responsibly be with more than one person. And some people love to happily remain solo. Any of these situations can be true for straight, gay, lesbian, bisexual, pansexual, or any other sexual orientation. If any of us wants to have physical intimacy, we all figure out how to use body parts and other fun tools and toys we can acquire, regardless of our identity.

ATTRACTION and IDENTITY do *not* predict BEHAVIOR.

So Dad, given that "greedy" is a behavior, when it comes to me being a bisexual woman, I'm no more or less gluttonous than my straight siblings, thank you very much!

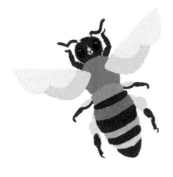

Which Label Is Better, Bisexual or Pansexual?

12

This is a *fabulous* question, especially for the queer community.

Let's start from scratch and consider how someone knows that they are straight. I used to think I was straight. In fact, I was straight. Not because I was smothering any feelings towards people of the same gender as me—hell, I made out with a few of my university girlfriends, kissing them in front of the lads (that's guys, y'all)—but never even considered I might not be straight. I mean, most of us are raised to be straight, and LGBTQIA+ people simply weren't visible to me during the 1990s. I knew I was straight because I was attracted to guys. End of story.

Then in my mid-20s, I had the opportunity to make out with a couple of friends who were girls, and this time it was different. The experience was undeniably hot, hot, hot. So at 27 years old, I came flying out of the closet as a lesbian. I knew I was a woman. I was attracted to women. Therefore, I completely overlooked the "B" in LGBT and labeled myself lesbian or gay, just

like films and TV shows typically and inconsiderately do. Simple as that.

Or so I thought. Eight years later, I found myself dating guys again on the down-low, which felt riskier than dating a woman. I'd made a name for myself as a lesbian, so I was anxious that my queer friends would call me a fraud and accuse me of not being gay enough. But when I was honest with myself, I realized that the only reason I had been turning down dates with men was because I'd told myself that I was gay.

When I figured out that bisexual was more accurate, I felt like I was losing an identity that had become such a integral piece of my being. But the great news was that I shared an identity with over 50 percent of the lesbian, gay, and bisexual (LGB) community. Yup! Statistically over half of LGB people say "bisexual" when asked in an anonymous survey.[1] It's just that too many people are afraid to say it publicly because the stigma is rampant, so our label has remained dreadfully disregarded for too long. But you watch. Things are changing quickly.

In 2012 I finally embraced my position as a B within LGBT and came out as bisexual on YouTube™. These days, my video is old school compared to today's cool and efficient TikTok® posts featuring bisexuals who are unable to sit still, some sporting cuffed jeans, and a few more with

clear iPhone® cases, but I got some lovely comments and one said I described myself as pansexual.

I'll take that as a compliment given that bisexuals have mistakenly been thought to only be attracted to cisgender men or cisgender women—whereas most bisexual people, myself included, see beyond that binary.

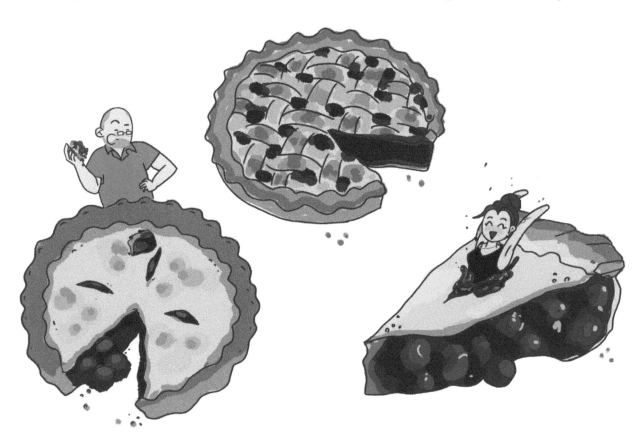

♥ Fiona and her dad, Peter, enjoying different pieces of cherry pie. ♥

"Bi" means "two." Therefore bisexuals have the capacity to be attracted to the same gender, or a different gender. As in a gender different from their own.

"Pan" means "all." Therefore pansexuals have the capacity to be attracted to all genders.

Lemme ask y'all a question:

Who likes cherries?

I dare to say that most people have enjoyed eating a cherry or two in their time. But did you know that there are more than 1,000 varieties of cherries grown in the United States, and not all of them taste the same?[2] Within the two categories of sweet and sour there's a whole spectrum of different cherries with different nuances, colors, expressions, flavors and so on. But they're all still cherries.

Now, imagine for a minute that cherries represent genders.

Bing cherries are the variety typically used in pie. Let's say straight people only eat bing cherry pie. They don't like *every* bing cherry pie they come across. Some like more crust, some less. Some like lattice, some like a lid. But in general, when asked, straight people say they like bing cherry pie and would not consume any other cherry in pie or in another form.

Bisexual people like bing cherry pie too. Like straight people, they don't all want every bing cherry pie, but they're definitely attracted to bing cherry pie.

However, unlike straight people, they're also open to enjoying a pie made with a different cherry varietal. And not all bisexual people are the same:

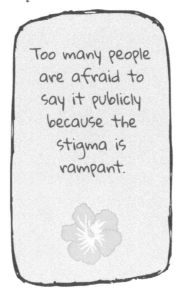

Too many people are afraid to say it publicly because the stigma is rampant.

Some bisexual people like bing cherry pie and one other cherry varietal.

Some bisexual people like bing cherry pie and more than one other cherry varietal.

Some bisexual people like bing cherry pie and many other cherry varietals.

Some bisexual people like bing cherry pie and they've no idea how many other cherry varietals because there are so many to choose from and how could they possibly know if they haven't tried them all? They may like all the cherries or they may only like a few, but they certainly don't want to limit their options.

Pansexual people like bing cherry pie and potentially all other cherry pies.

So is bisexual or pansexual better? It depends on who's asking. If you're labeling yourself, the answer is whichever label feels better for you. If you're labeling someone else, then just don't. Don't label someone else. Politely ask them how they identify and accept their reply. Period.

Now, where's that pie?

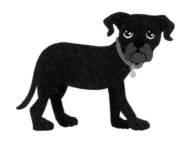

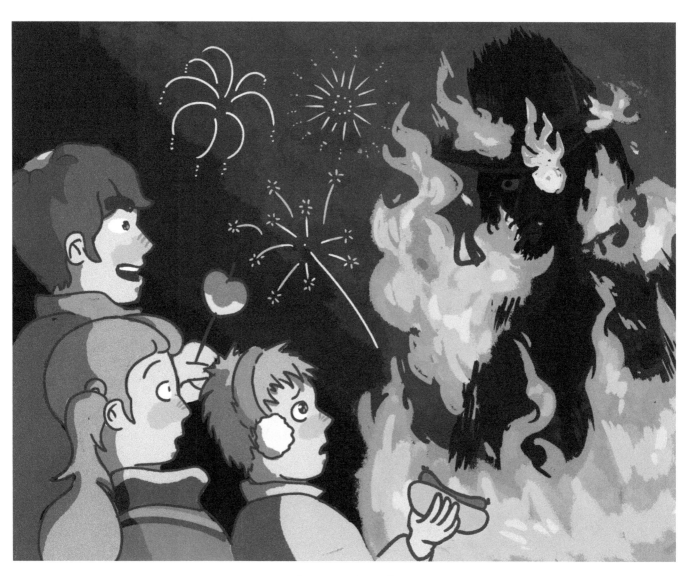

♥ Fiona's siblings Joey and Rob at Bonfire Night with their dad. ♥

Why Are We Saying, "Hey Guys!" to Greet Women?

13

I know this one is *really* going to ruffle some feathers, including among my friends, but I have to just put it out there.

You've probably figured out by now that I don't like to lump people into one of two buckets, and I think it's extremely important to call people by their correct name and pronouns. Most of my friends, of *all* political persuasions, would agree with me on this. So why on earth "Hey guys!" has become such an accepted greeting when there are women in the room absolutely baffles me. In fact, I'm a member of various friend circles with only women and they excitedly hail each other with, "Hey guys!" and in my mind it's like nails on a chalkboard.

This is not an exclusively cultural thing as all across the world, including in the UK, people say, "Hey guys!" to greet a mix of people. YouTube reports that "Hey guys!" accounts for 36 percent of the top five greetings creators use to start their vlogs. But even YouTube states that this raises " ... gender inclusivity questions we won't get into here."[1]

What shocks me the most are my liberal, feminist friends calling each other guys. The original definition of guy is "man." Nothing against men, but as a woman, I don't want my identity to be melted into a man's. Think of all the other terms that are rooted in masculine language that we should also be changing: chairman, congressman, freshman, fireman, milkman, mailman. Mankind. All men are created equal. And don't even get me started on the sign, "Men at Work." If we're creating gender equity in the world, then why are we continuing to use this male-centered language?

As a British-American I particularly resonate with the source of the word "guy," and here's the story as to why:

As a child my friends and I would recite the nursery rhyme,

"Remember, remember, the Fifth of November

Gunpowder treason and plot

I see no reason why gunpowder treason

Should ever be forgot."

From as early as I can remember, on the evening of November 5th my parents would take us to the local rugby club, where the players had constructed a massive bonfire with a stuffed scarecrow of a man burning in the middle. There would be a hot dog stand, our hands would freeze beneath our mittens, and we'd crane our necks into the cold, dark sky to watch an explosion of fantastic fireworks. The whole event would scare the shit out of my younger sister, Joey (she/her), so invariably she'd hide under Dad's coat. My younger brother, Rob (he/him), just gazed up with wide-open starry eyes. I was a little creeped out by the burning effigy, but the hot dog and sparklers were enough to keep me happy.

The stuffed figure in flames resembled Guy Fawkes (he/him), who orchestrated a failed attempt to blow up the Houses of Parliament on November 5th, 1605. Given his goal was the equivalent of trying to blow up the US Capitol with a full House, Senate, and President inside, Fawkes and his co-conspirators were sentenced to death with the brutal British order of being hung, drawn, and quartered. This literally describes what they would do to his body, so Fawkes wisely jumped before this torture could be implemented and died of a broken neck.[2]

In celebration of the plot failing and King James I (he/him) surviving, the Brits burned bonfires and ignited fireworks to happy cheers.[3] And like many traditions, with the addition of a hot dog stand, the annual ritual continues to the present day.

But the failed attempt to blow up Parliament, *which happened over 400 years ago when women were still property*, ignited not just bonfires, but the use of the word "guy" to imply a poorly dressed, male-presenting person. I distinctly remember when I was a kid growing up in the UK, passing a pair of teenagers sitting outside the chemist shop with their model of Fawkes to be burned that night, peddling with the words, "Penny for the guy! Penny for the guy!"

Since the gunpowder, treason, and plot of 1605, the term was carried across the world, with colonialism of course, and today we find people of all genders, including women, jumping onto calls and excitedly greeting with, "Hey guys!"[4]

Given I'm not a guy, i.e. a poorly dressed male-presenting person, I can't help but feel excluded by this greeting, no matter how well-meaning it is. And if *I* feel like that, I can only imagine how a gender nonbinary person feels. Or a trans woman who has had to

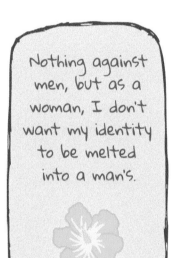

Nothing against men, but as a woman, I don't want my identity to be melted into a man's.

fake being a "guy" for years before courageously coming out. For these reasons, I'm practicing only using this word to greet people I know identify as male, and I'll even include those who dress well.

How about the next time you're on a group call with one or more men present, you try greeting them with, "Hey gals!" and see what happens. Or maybe, just say "Hey y'all!" Because if this British-born, posh-accented, American immigrant can say "y'all," then all of y'all can too! ;)

Or should I just get over it and join the bandwagon of saying, "Hey guys!"?

I guess change does happen. But ... Nails. On. A. Chalkboard.

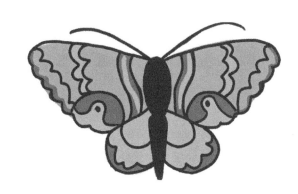

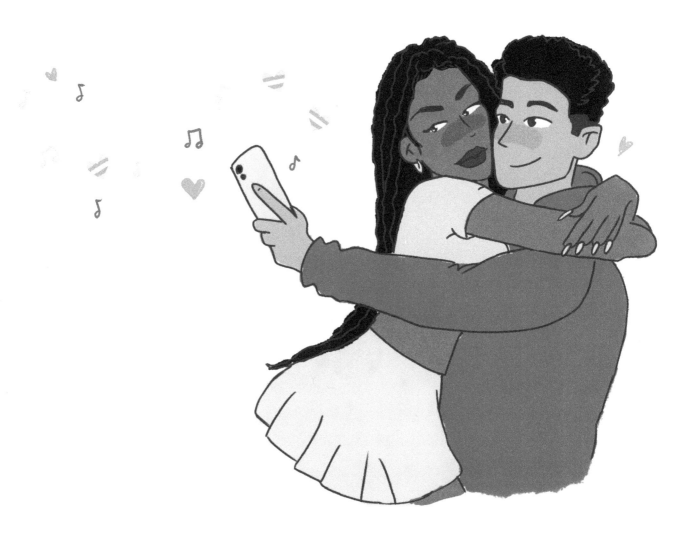

♥ The fierce and adorable social media power couple
Jayde McFarlane @jaydemcfarlane and Tyler Lyons @ty.13.r.lyons. ♥

If a Straight Man Wants to Make Love with a Transgender Woman, Does It Mean He's Gay? 14

The quick answer to this is no. It does not make him gay. Sexual orientation is a personal and internal identity, and not created on the basis of the biological sex and/or gender of the person you're attracted to.

I think some people get confused about this because we focus on the wrong part of our bodies. We're so fixated with what's between someone's legs, which is very personal, that we're overlooking what's wired in our brains.

As I explained in Chapter 11, all human beings have three different components to our sexual orientation:

♥ Number one: our ATTRACTION. This is who you want to go to bed with.

Attraction is our capacity for love, romance, and/or sexual feelings towards others determined by our genes and hormones, i.e. wired into our brains. Some of the attraction is determined by the gender you're attracted to and some by the genitals you're attracted to. And this is on a different scale for different people, and at different times. Some people experience attraction and some people don't. Like practically everything in life, it's on a spectrum.

♥ Number two: our IDENTITY. This is who you go to bed as.

This is the sexual orientation and gender labels we give to ourselves based on who we're attracted to when compared to our own gender. This is who we know ourselves to be. It's how we're wired and it's not a choice.

Most people are straight, meaning that they have the capacity to be attracted to someone of a different gender than their own. Some people are not straight, meaning that they have the capacity to be attracted to someone of a different gender and/or same gender as their own.

Oftentimes straight and not straight people are attracted to others before we have any idea what their genitals look like! And we may never know what they look like given it's not our freaking business.

45

Most women are born with female genitalia, but some women are born with male genitalia. Most men are born with male genitalia, but some men are born with female genitalia. And some people are intersex, meaning that they have any combination of male and female sex tissue, chromosomes, and/or hormones. But it's your *gender* that makes you a woman, a man, or any other identity, and **not** your genitals!

♥   Number three: our BEHAVIOR. This is what you would like to do in bed. Or in a shower, car, park bench, or anywhere else that tickles your fancy ;). And sometimes it's just sleeping!

Behavior is how we act upon our attraction and identity. Many people implement their love, romance, and/or sexual feelings with one person, some

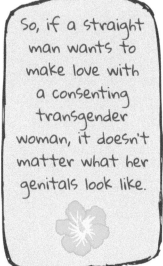

So, if a straight man wants to make love with a consenting transgender woman, it doesn't matter what her genitals look like.

people implement these feelings with more than one person, and some people love to happily remain solo.

But you see, our genitals are *not* the organs making any of the decisions here. In the same way a hand doesn't decide how the artist will draw, our genitals don't decide how we'll make love. It's the brain that sees the beautiful canvas and guides in painting the pretty picture.

So, if a straight man wants to make love with a consenting transgender woman, it doesn't matter what *her* genitals look like. That's private information between the adoring couple and none of our freaking business!

And quite frankly, we don't accuse our heterosexual, cisgender neighbors of turning gay if they have a little anal play, so all this judging of who people are based upon gender and genitals is quite ridiculous!

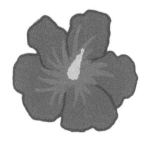

Do All Transgender Men Want Male Genitalia?

15

Nope.

You gotta admit, this is a really rather personal and direct question.

First of all there are many cisgender guys out there who would like to amend the appearance, and maybe function, of their genitalia too. Given the US military annually spends $84.24 million dollars on erectile dysfunction prescriptions,[1] there are a helluva lot of dudes out there who need a little pick me up, shall we say. And when you combine reports on the number of deployed US service members sustaining injury to their genitals in war zones[2] with the global count of penis enlargements last reported in 2013 by the International Society of Aesthetic Plastic Surgery being 15,000,[3, 4] it seems that cisgender men get phalloplasty—aka a medically constructed penis—more often than transgender men.

But you know what? Let's not make this a pissing competition as no one should be shamed for the make or model of their body, or how it functions.

All people deserve access to the medical care they need. It's a human right. Including those cisgender dudes in the military and including all transgender people.

One of the humps we need to get over is this false notion that a man is defined by having male genitalia and a woman is defined by having female genitalia.

There are many problematic issues with this, but the most striking to me is that this theory completely overlooks the existence of intersex people.

As I've mentioned a few times now, one in 100 Americans are born intersex, meaning that they have any variation of sex tissue, chromosomes, and/or hormones. For comparison's sake, one in 100 Americans are also born with red hair.

Stop and think: how many people do you know who have naturally red hair?

I can think of my childhood friend Lizzie (she/her), one of my besties Chris (he/him), a fantastic ex-boyfriend who took me on some incredible vacations, Emil (he/him), and my mum.

Although hers faded over time. Don't tell anyone, but my red hair is "applied" ;). So without knowing, because I don't see *all* of my friend's genitals, that's roughly the number of intersex people I've probably been close to in my life. Not to mention the other thousands I've passed on the street.

But let's get back to the spectrum of genitals. There are several intersex people sharing their lived experience in an educational way online. Someone who I greatly admire is Alicia Roth Weigel (she/her), who has a fantastic memoir titled *Inverse Cowgirl.* Alicia's story and bold activism is educational and motivating.

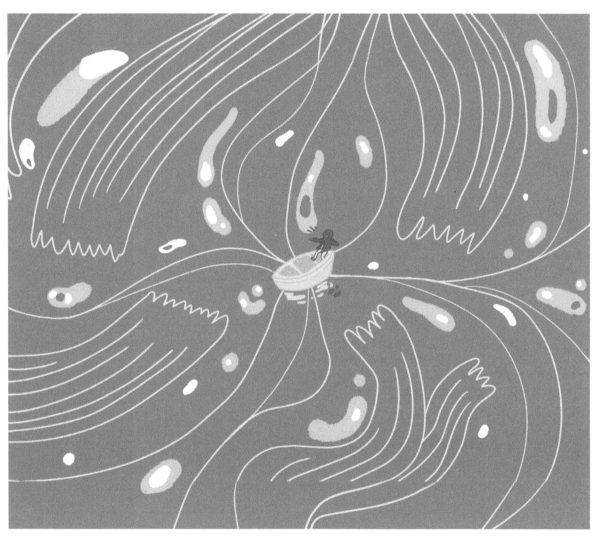

♥ Dysphoria. ♥

There are many variations possible within an intersex person's body, but in a nutshell, someone could be born with visible male genitalia and also have ovaries like a cisgender woman and XY chromosomes. Or, visible female genitalia and also testes like a cisgender man and XX chromosomes. But you should really go check out Alicia's book and Pidgeon Pigonis's (they/them) YouTube channel as they explain their personal story so smartly—including the savage decision of doctors to conduct surgery when they were four years old. Savage.

What intersex people help us directly understand is that sex tissue, chromosomes, and hormones do not predict gender. Gender is absolutely something that is wired in our brains, can be fluid over time, and is influenced by society. It's not defined by our genitals. And gender is on a spectrum.

When a transgender man, who is someone born with female genitalia or is intersex and was labeled as a woman, comes to understand that they are a man, they can consider whether their body feels comfortable the way it is, or if having medical treatment is necessary to stop feelings of *dysphoria*.

"What's dysphoria?" I hear you ask. Given I'm cisgender and haven't experienced dysphoria I'm going to let my editor, Gus (he/him), take over and explain this one as he's trans and has had firsthand experience.

Hey Gus!

Hey Fiona!

I will now explain how dysphoria feels in the most dude way ever ...

Imagine you and all your friends own PlayStations®, and an eagerly anticipated game has just been released. Let's make it Dragon Age or Mass Effect, since Bioware™ has awesome queer representation, yay!

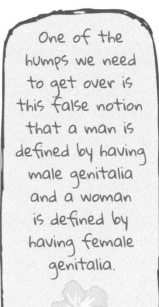

One of the humps we need to get over is this false notion that a man is defined by having male genitalia and a woman is defined by having female genitalia.

Anyway, everyone picks up their copy and takes it home to play on their PlayStations. As a trans person with dysphoria, it feels like you were mistakenly given the Xbox version of the game—you just want to play and have fun like everyone else, but in order to do so, you need to go through a series of extra steps.

And of course, people who know nothing about game systems can't understand why you aren't happy with what you were given. Isn't it the same game? It has the same cover art. But. It. Does. Not. Work. You are still left out. You can't participate until you get the copy of the game that works in your game system. And having to wait to get the right version while everyone else has fun is pretty crappy.

So that's how I'd best describe dysphoria.

Back to you, Fiona.

Thanks, Gus! I love that analogy.

I've heard different friends describe dysphoria in different ways. One friend told me it's like being trapped on a boat out on a rough sea and you have no way of getting your bearings, but everyone else seems to be walking steadily on dry land.

It sounds like getting the right version of the game like Gus described helps the world to make sense. But getting the right version can be different things for different people. I know that starting with hormones to reach the right balance can help some people.

Surgery can also help, but not all transgender people need surgery to affirm their gender. Lemme state this again: Not all transgender people need or want surgery. Some people do not feel like they were "born in the wrong body" and are quite happy to keep things as they are,[5] thank you very much!

As with everything in life, people's feelings about their bodies fall on a spectrum. Some transgender men and transmasculine people decide that having a penis removes or decreases their dysphoria. Some decide that they don't have that dysphoric feeling from not having a penis, and they'd rather keep their genitals exactly as they are. Some might occasionally benefit from a prosthetic penis (like a packer or STP, which I'll describe further in the next chapter) but not surgery, especially because medical science still has a long way to go in perfecting genital surgeries. It is typically extremely painful, leaves scar tissue where skin has been grafted, and does not always produce the ultimate desired results. And some other people may make other personal and private decisions about their body parts that are absolutely none of our business, just like cisgender people do.

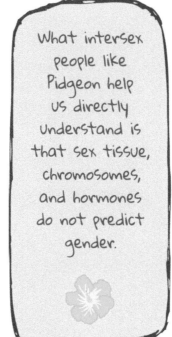

What intersex people like Pidgeon help us directly understand is that sex tissue, chromosomes, and hormones do not predict gender.

The bottom line here is that some men have female genitalia and some women have male genitalia. And some people have a combination of the two. Just like there are more than two makes of cars in the world, there are more than two ways genitals are designed.

The most important point is that every person should feel comfortable within the human body they are living in, so they can play the game and be at peace on dry land just like everyone else.

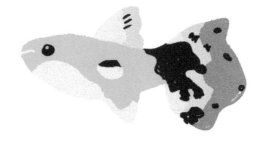

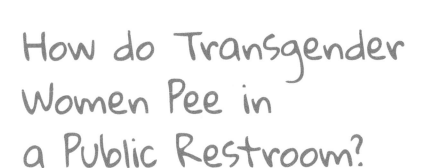

How do Transgender Women Pee in a Public Restroom?

16

First of all it's none of our freaking business how transgender women, or anyone for that matter, pee in a public restroom. But given there's a lack of understanding, I thought I better explain a thing or two.

Let's imagine a person who identifies as a woman walks into the female restroom. If there are no stalls available, they patiently wait. A stall becomes available, they go in, lock the door, and typically sit down to pee. Where no one can see.

Once finished, they wisely wash their hands, maybe adjust their hair, and re-apply some lipstick, and get on with their day.

It's as simple as that. Or at least it should be.

You see, my trans friends are fearful about whether they can get in, do their business, and get out of the restroom without getting beaten up. So much so that they'll train themselves to hold it for eight hours or more, which has terrible health consequences. And some of my other friends think that trans women are men in dresses who want to assault little girls.

And I love all of y'all, so let's bridge this gap.

We need to remember that you can't tell what someone's genitals look like simply by judging their gender. Gender is wired in our brains whereas our genitals are between our legs. Some women are born with male genitalia, and some men are born with female genitalia. And one in 100 people born in the United States are intersex, meaning that they have any variation of male and female sex tissue, chromosomes, and/or hormones.

Because we typically don't walk around naked, we actually have no idea what most people's genitals look like. And it's really none of our business.

It also makes giving people one of two choices of where to relieve themselves a little nonsensical, especially when there are more than two variations of genitals. Most public restrooms are saying if you have male genitalia go in here, where we also have urinals, and if you have female genitalia go in here, where we don't include urinals.

But what if you have a combination of male genitalia and female genitalia? Then where does society expect you to go? And while men's restrooms have stalls too, the implication is that men stand, and I know many cisgender dudes with male genitalia who like to pee sitting down. And many transgender dudes with female genitalia who like to piss standing up.

Standing up to pee with a vagina without getting urine all over yourself is possible, and quite an art without assistance. I unsuccessfully tried when I was a kid because I wanted to see what it was like. I straddled the toilet facing the tank, barely tall enough to hover over the bowl. It must've been quite a sight for the fly on the wall. Today, I could purchase a special funnel which would be quite handy on a camping trip, and trans guys have the option of getting an "STP," which is the acronym for "Stand To Pee."

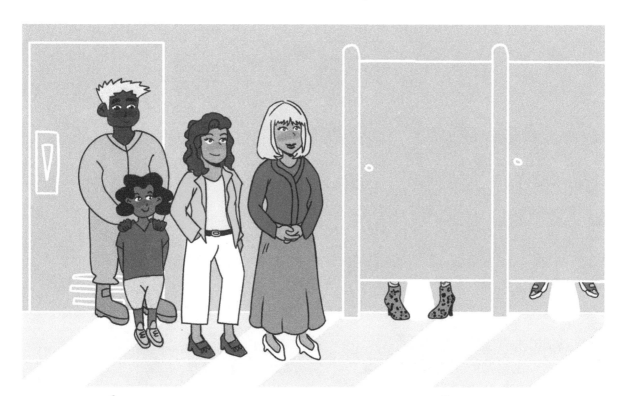

♥ Fiona's friends Sheila and Mindy patiently wait for a toilet stall. ♥

An STP is a prosthetic device that can medically stick to the body or be held in place with customized underwear. They come in all shapes and sizes, including as a prosthetic penis. Individuals who feel more comfortable having a penis and wish to stand to pee like cisgender guys can choose to wear them and pee where cis dudes pee.

Just like cisgender females in the women's restroom, many cisgender males in the men's room have probably peed next to a trans person and had absolutely no idea. Those cis guys went in and came out of the restroom like it was no big deal, but those trans guys may have been shaking in their boots hoping that not only did they not piss all over themselves, but someone didn't realize they were born with female genitalia and decide to punch them for it.

At the end of the day, just because someone's gender expression or body parts don't match what society says a man or a woman should look like, it doesn't mean that they pee any differently than anyone else. They either sit, squat, or stand. What we all have in common is that we would like to relieve ourselves safely and privately in a clean toilet.

When studies show that there are *zero* reports of a transgender person in the United

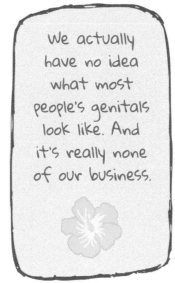

We actually have no idea what most people's genitals look like. And it's really none of our business.

States assaulting someone in a public restroom,[1] but transgender people are four times more likely to *be* assaulted,[2] regardless of our gender and our genitals, the greatest risks we *all* face are from those people who don't wash their hands!

So when presented with a "male" sign or a "female" sign, ask yourself if you're being policed on what's in your pants or how you're expressing your gender to the world. And maybe you'll come to agree that restrooms should be single-stall private potties where any person is free to pee or poop in peace!

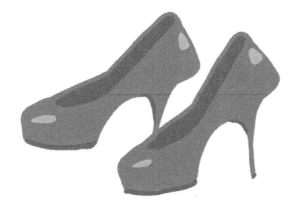

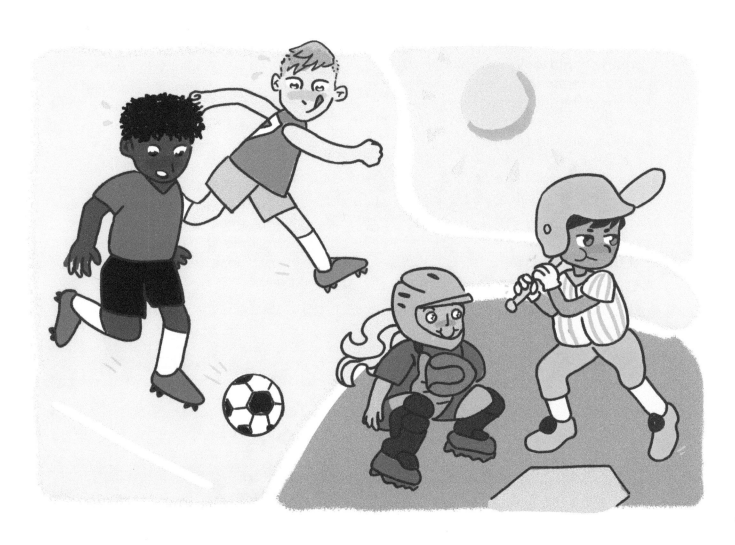

♥ Fiona's nephew Oscar plays football with his friends. ♥

Why Does Allowing Athletes who are Transgender to Compete in School Sports Make America Great?

17

There were some epic athletic wins for women back in the "before times" of 2019. Not to mention a freaking legendary display of joyful teammate camaraderie by the Auburn Women's Basketball Team in their locker room dance-off to Lil Wayne's "Uproar." It went viral, so it's an easy search.

When it comes to getting awards, UCLA gymnast Katelyn Ohashi (she/her) thrilled us with a perfect ten at the 2019 Collegiate Challenge, we gave massive respect for twenty-two-year-old Simone Biles (she/her) becoming the most decorated athlete in history, and we felt national pride when the US Women's Soccer team won the Women's World Cup ... again!

Yet, as I write this, seven US states have banned transgender kids from playing school sports and around 20 more are trying, saying trans girls will "ruin women's sports." Oops. I haven't even finished editing and it's now up to eight.[1]

Ummm ... what the freaking frig? It makes no sense. Transgender athletes have been *openly* playing in high school and college sports since 2008.[2] So given all of these (presumably) cisgender women's successes, it doesn't seem like their participation has been that "disruptive" to me.

In fact, transgender people have been playing sports on this planet for as long as any other human beings have been playing sports on this planet. Transgender people have always existed.

At first blush, I can understand why a well-meaning person would think that transgender girls have an advantage over cisgender girls, but when you take a step back and learn the facts, it's easy to see why our first assumption is not based on science or biology. It's based on stereotypes.

You see, some people think that trans women and girls have strong male bodies and will knock out their competition. And trans men and boys ... well, they're not even considered because clearly they're just physically weak, like women and girls. Because *all* men are strong and *all* women are weak, right?

I'm being sarcastic, btw.

The fact is, none of this is true. If it were, then even though transgender athletes have been allowed to compete in the Olympics since 2004,[3] why did it take another 17 years for any openly trans* athletes to actually qualify? Chris Mosier (he/him) competed in the 2020 trials but had to withdraw due to an injury.[4] In 2021 three athletes who are transgender qualified for Tokyo, including Canadian soccer player Quinn (they/them), who made history by becoming the first openly transgender, nonbinary athlete to win an Olympic gold medal. Whoop, whoop! But no other athletes who are transgender—especially note that this includes those assigned male at birth—have won any Olympic medals. Ever.[5] And at the time of this book going to print, not one openly trans* athlete has won the Heisman. Or Wimbledon. Or the Super Bowl. Need I go on? Unfair advantage my ass. Gah.

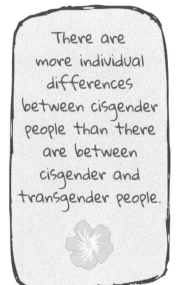

There are more individual differences between cisgender people than there are between cisgender and transgender people.

You see, we're still a little confused on biology. As I've said before, some women are born with male genitalia and some men are born with female genitalia. And some people are intersex meaning that they have any combination of male and female sex tissue, chromosomes, and/or hormones.

But not one human being—cisgender, transgender, or intersex—is born with identical hormonal levels or physical bodies. Cisgender people naturally have varying hormonal levels and physical characteristics. We're all beautifully unique and have an opportunity to use our bodies within the range of our physical selves. It's how *athletic* we are that leads to success, not whether we're cisgender or transgender.

There are more individual differences between cisgender people than there are between cisgender and transgender people.[6] Think about it. Is every woman the same? Is every man the same?

I've been a curvy, five-foot-one-with-larger-than-average-ass-and-thighs female since before puberty. For seven years I swam for my home town, training up to six times a week. My friend of the same age, Samantha (she/her), had the same training schedule as me and *always* beat me in races. Okay, maybe I beat her once and cried with glorious shock. Anyway, Sam was a tall, slender, strong swimmer and probably had a more determined mental attitude than me too. Overall, she was simply a better swimmer. Neither of us are trans, btw.

Even those lawmakers who claim cisgender girls are pushed out of sports, are having their records beaten, are losing out on scholarships, and basically have been made to feel less-than, **cannot name one single instance of when this has happened.[7]**

On the flip side, when trans girls at puberty have life-saving—yes, literally life-saving—medical treatment, they have no physical advantage over cis, or non-transgender, girls. Before life-saving medical treatment—like puberty blockers—they are very unlikely to participate in sports due to bullying, stigma, and discrimination. But even then, their bodies aren't necessarily more athletic. We simply don't see transgender girls or boys playing with a physical advantage. If anything, trans* kids have to train harder than cis kids to win.[8]

But it's not just about winning, is it?

We know that playing sports has countless positive effects on human beings—that's one of the reasons why America is consumed with so many sporting pastimes, which makes me wonder why no known trans people have made it into Major League Baseball. Oh yeah. Stigma. I digress.

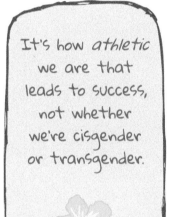

It's how *athletic* we are that leads to success, not whether we're cisgender or transgender.

The truth is, when transgender youth are included along with the 60 percent of kids that participate in a sport,[9] more girls are happily playing sports together, celebrating each other's wins and helping each other improve their skills. The joyful sense of community, courage, and confidence that comes from playing sports can literally save transgender and cisgender kids' lives.[10, 11]

I know that's definitely the case for my friends who have a 14-year-old daughter who's trans. Only people on a need-to-know basis know she was assigned male at birth. Everyone else assumes she's cis. But she's running track with her friends, has a massive smile on her face, and is not winning. Just like every other kid who doesn't finish first.

Because we teach kids it's the participation that counts. Right?

I have another thought … Why are we grouping people based upon their genitals in the first place? Doesn't it wrongly assume that all girls are not as athletic as all boys?

When I was in the swim club of my home town in Boston, UK, we had an A squad and a B squad based upon your speed. I was typically in the B squad with my friend Dale (he/him), who is a boy (presumably cisgender), as we often got similar times. Whereas Sam, who is the cisgender girl I mentioned above, would whip both of us and make it into the A squad. So wouldn't it make more sense for humans to compete and be scored within similar athletic ability rather than by biological sex or gender? The US Army is already doing this with their "Army Combat Fitness Test."[12]

So, as we come to understand that gender and genitals exist on a spectrum and have little to do with our athletic ability, let's be more concerned about rich parents bribing coaches to admit their kids to college—or stopping body shaming gymnasts like Ohashi with her perfect 10, or celebrating equal pay for women soccer players—rather than needlessly obsessing over if some kids aren't meeting society's expectation of gender.

When we support *all* youth to train hard, build their self-esteem, and feel that they belong, we will not only make America great. We'll make the world great.

P.S. Watch the documentary *Changing the Game*. It's awesome, you'll see.

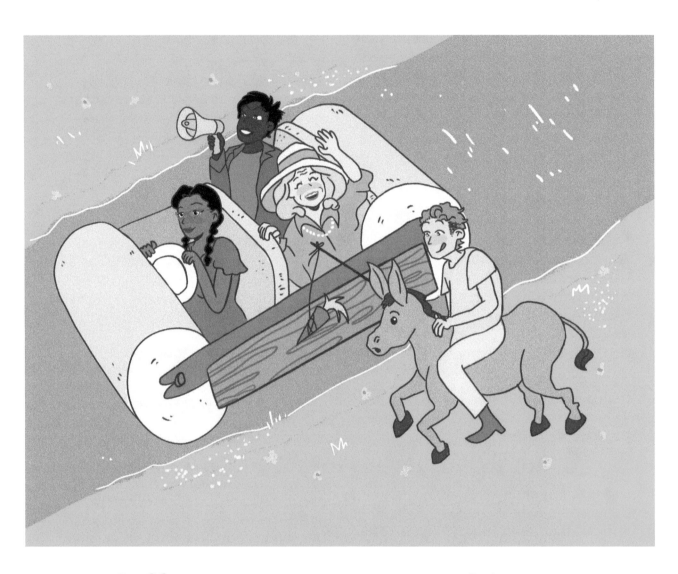

♥ Raffi Freedman-Gurspan drives Monica Roberts and
Edie Windsor, while Chris McNeany rides his donkey to the office. ♥

Why Can't I Love the Sinner but Hate the Sin?

18

There was once a time when I was a good little practicing Catholic girl. Growing up we'd say prayers every night, I'd get on my knees every Sunday morning in church, and regularly went to confession to rid myself of all my wretched sins. Although it was super hard to think of what to admit to the priest sometimes. My first confession at the age of seven was that I'd eaten a ton of sweets at the school party when my mum had specifically told me not to. As you can tell, I was a very naughty girl.

But living to the dictates of God was extremely important to me as I didn't want to go to Hell. I read my children's Bible from start to finish *twice* and believed that there was never a reason for an abortion. As for gay people, well, I didn't even know that they existed, so their place in the Catholic church wasn't even a consideration to me.

And then in my 20s, I came out as a lesbian. Now I heard "Love the sinner, hate the sin," but I knew I was no more of a sinner than I'd been at any

other time of my life. And the biggest takeaway I'd gotten from the Bible was to love everyone, especially people who were different from me in some way.

So while I respect people of all or no faiths, I have people in my life who claim their dedication to Christianity, but while they say they love me as a friend, they also fear that LGBTQIA+ people, myself included, are going to Hell. They're still afraid, like I was, that God will punish me because the Bible says I'm wrong.

Well, I love those friends back and want to relieve their fear and let them know that in fact the Bible doesn't say us queers are going to Hell. And here's why:

♥ The Bible is really, really, really freaking old. I mean super old. Like the Old Testament is between 3,220 and 2,185 years old. Remember the cartoon *The Flintstones*? That's what the UK would've looked like when they were writing it back then. Didn't they also think the world was flat?

♥ The New Testament was written during the first 100 years after the

59

birth of Jesus, so we're talking around 1,920 years old. People didn't have words for "straight," let alone "gay" back then. There wasn't a concept of homosexuality. Going back to prehistoric times, people were sexually engaged with each other regardless of what their genitals looked like, but they didn't label it.[1]

♥ The original Bible was not written in English. It was written in three languages: Hebrew, Aramaic, and Greek. It's hard enough to translate Shakespeare's 400-year-old English into our modern-day understanding, let alone Hebrew, Aramaic, and Greek from thousands of years ago! Although some researchers are now saying that from analyzing his words, Shakespeare was bisexual, and I'm certainly not going to argue that one![2]

♥ Imagine the Bible's authors writing the following paragraph in their language:

"The second gentleman and his wife, Madam Vice-President, had a blast creating viral TikTok videos in their pod during the pandemic, but the idea to turn them into a miniseries got a hard pass when pitched to Netflix™."

Impossible. And just like second gentlemen, viral TikTok videos, a pod in a pandemic, and passes from Netflix, (all terms just added to the Merriam-Webster dictionary, btw) the concept of homosexuality just didn't exist.[3]

> People didn't have words for "straight," let alone "gay" back then.

♥ So let's move on to those six or seven (depending on how you count) places out of the 66 books or 1,200 pages that make up the library we call "the Bible" that supposedly address homosexuality. There's actually a fantastic documentary y'all should watch called *For the Bible Tells Me So*, which addresses every single one.

Spoiler alert: the translation of the thousands-of-years-old language from back when people were still riding their donkeys to the office, is slightly off.

Here's a brief, *very* basic, breakdown:[4]

♥ The story of Sodom and Gomorrah (Genesis 19) = Rape. Rape's never good.

♥ The Book of Leviticus (18:22 and 20:13) = Make babies, we need them to keep society growing. Adoption and artificial insemination hadn't been invented yet. Side note: Leviticus also bans tattoos, pork, shellfish, gives rules for selling a slave, and says all foreigners must be welcomed into your country. I told you, stuff changes with time!

♥ 1 Corinthians (6:9-10) and 1 Timothy (1:10) = If you're a man, don't be like a woman. You know, all soft, sensitive, and taking it in a nondominant position ... and maneuvers like that. Because that's clearly what all women do. And you older men shouldn't treat the younger ones like crap. Have some respect, for goodness' sake.

♥ Romans (1:26-27) = Don't have sex just for fun. Especially women, who get a first mention here, btw. Dude, sex is for making babies and women need to stay passive and in their place, especially during sex. Calm down with that passion, y'all.

Again, thousands of years later, human beings have become a little more worldly and wise. At least for the most part.

A slight slip happened on February 11, 1946, when the word "homosexual" was mistakenly entered into the Bible for the first time.[5] A bunch of guys translated some Greek all wrong, and experts now agree the word used should've been something like "pervert" instead. I used to barely pass my high school Greek classes because understanding other languages can be hard, but the consequences of this mistranslation have caused major pain and suffering around the world. The director of *For the Bible Tells Me So* is now executive producer on a new film, *1946: The Mistranslation That Shifted a Culture,* to teach us all about the word homosexuality being added to the Bible, and I can't wait to watch!

> A slight slip happened on February 11, 1946, when the word "homosexual" was mistakenly entered into the Bible for the first time.

But as a reminder of our present day, we now drive around in cars powered by engines rather than with our feet like *The Flintstones*. We have birth control. We realize that sexual relationships—like everything else in life—exist on a spectrum. Some people do want to have sex, some people want it sometimes, and some people don't at all. And our capacity for attraction is as vastly diverse as an ocean bed. If you've read the previous chapters, you'll catch my drift.

For those that believe these men's (no women or anyone with another gender is recorded as authoring any of the Bible) words are directly words of God, when you read perspective from experts who are much smarter than me and have dedicated their lives to studying the Bible, they agree that the writings are opinion, anecdotes, and personal stories. Things we can read to gather inspiration from rather than always literally believe. Kinda like a few other publications out there ;)

Regardless to what degree we take the Bible as gospel, I truly feel that our calling in life is to center in Love. Yes, Love with a capital L. We live in a magical, beautiful world created by Spirit with whichever name is best for you. Mine is God or the Universe, and I see and feel this Spirit everywhere.

Have you seen the 2021 Best Documentary Oscar-winning film, *My Octopus Teacher,* about a man who forms a relationship with an octopus? Their bond illustrates the perfect spiritual connection that all living creatures have the capacity to feel together in this world.

The octopus's environment within the water is a whole different ecosystem, existing every day alongside ours, that virtually none of us ever get to see. It's another vibrant neighborhood filled with creatures simply surviving, to fulfill their purpose before they leave this physical realm and move onto the next. Just like all of us creatures here on land.

The fact is, like gender and genitals, God made sexual orientation on a spectrum. Birds and bees have same-gender lovin' relations. As do fish, dolphins, monkeys, elephants, giraffes, goats, pandas, and on and on.[6, 7] I guess not reading the Bible helped these animals freely express themselves.

I don't want to take the Bible away from anyone who wants to keep it, but I can't help but think how wonderful it would be if out of all the words to cling onto *literally* in the text, we selected Matthew 22:39.

"Thou shalt love thy neighbour as thyself."

Well, that's the British version, I guess. The American would be:

"Thou shalt love thy neighbor as thyself."

Just love friends, please. When it comes to LGBTQIA+ people, there's no sin to hate.

Love always.

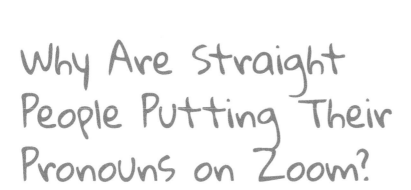

Why Are Straight People Putting Their Pronouns on Zoom?

19

Let me take you back to around 1987 to the small town in which I grew up. Y'all would call it a "city," but where I come from it's a "town" called Boston, situated about 100 miles north of London.

Yes, there's a Boston in England. And yes, London is not a country. It's the capital city of England, which is a country that along with Wales and Scotland form Great Britain. If you add Northern Ireland to that mix, you create the United Kingdom, and …

Gah, sorry, this is not a geography lesson but a bare-bones and binary explainer on pronouns. I'll stay on track.

I was about ten years old, and I wanted to model my mother *so* much that I had my hair cut super short just like hers. I have photos from that era where I look like my mother's mini-me.

One day, Mum and I went into the cobbler shop in Boston. Most of y'all are now thinking of delicious desserts, but in fact the other meaning of "cobbler" is someone who mends or makes shoes. Mum was dropping off a pair

and the friendly cobbler peered over his counter, looked down at little me and said,

"Now then, sonny! How are you?"

Calling a little boy "sonny" or "sonny Jim" is quite common in Britain, but I was immediately hurt and indignantly replied,

"I'm not a boy! I'm a girl!"

While I had that short hair, my gender was mistaken several times. I didn't know it back then, but the term we use today for this is *misgendered*. Friends of my parents who hadn't seen us for years would comment to Mum and Dad how lovely it was that they had two boys and a girl. They'd awkwardly correct that it was actually two girls and a boy.

I can still recall the deep distress I felt inside at being seen as a gender that I am not. Just imagine if I were that age living in America today, where at the time of me writing this in 2021, some lawmakers are suggesting that girls will have to show their private parts to adults before they can play sports.

That means I'd have to show I was assigned female at birth before competing on the swim team.[1]

You see, society has constructed its own rules, boxes, and expectations on how people are supposed to look and sound based upon more rules, boxes, and expectations covering only two genders. And all human minds are subconsciously making assumptions on who people are based upon how we see and hear them.

But gender identity and expression are *so* much more than just box A male and box B female. There exists a whole spectrum of ways people have been

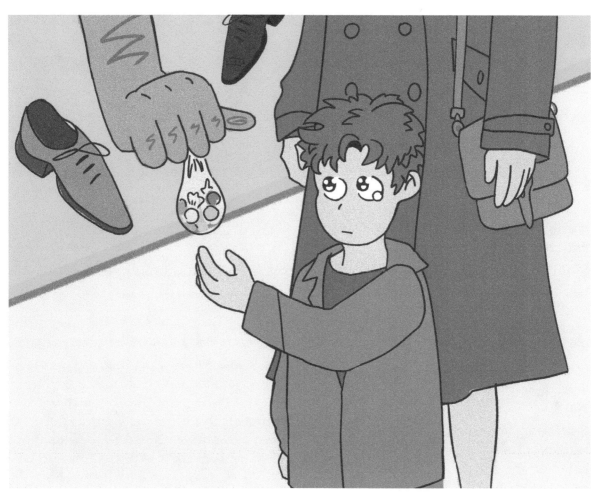

♥ Fiona with her mum accepting sweets from the cobbler. ♥

lovingly created to express how they feel on the inside. And there's nothing wrong with any of them. Some of us find it easier to fit into society's boxes than others, and that is a privilege as we don't even have to think about it. But I want to include and affirm people of *all* genders.

An easy yet profound way we can all help is to put our pronouns after our name whether we fit into a gender box or not. It says to everyone, "I'm an ally." It stops nonbinary and trans* people from being treated differently for stating their pronouns. And it helps everyone feel equally respected when being discussed.

The cobbler that day back in 1987 felt so bad for mistakenly calling me a boy, when Mum and I went back to pick up the shoes, he gave me a bag of sweets to apologize. I easily got over it. And now that I have long hair and present myself in a typically feminine conforming way, I don't get misgendered.

But for anyone who does not fit in a gender binary bucket (including straight, cisgender people), using correct pronouns literally saves lives.

Trigger warning:
The Trevor Project's *2021 National Survey on LGBTQ Youth Mental Health* reports, "Transgender and nonbinary youth who reported having pronouns respected by all of the people they lived with attempted suicide at half the rate of those who did not have their pronouns respected by anyone with whom they lived."[2]

That's a positive. *Only half* the rate if they're respected. It pains me to think of any young person wanting

An easy yet profound way we can all help is to put our pronouns after our name whether we fit into a gender box or not.

to die by suicide. Young people already face a ton of challenges in a changing world. Respect them with their correct pronouns please, for goodness' sake.

And if you are a young person considering suicide, please call the TrevorLifeline at 1-866-488-7386 or text "START" to 678-678 right now.

If you are over twenty-five years old and considering suicide, please call the National Suicide Prevention Lifeline at 1-800-273-8255 or text 988 right now.

Everyone else, please read on.

Today, let's together create a world where *all* people, of all ages, are respected. And that starts with gender-binary-presenting people of all sexual orientations putting their pronouns on Zoom too. And on Microsoft Teams. And on their email signature. And on their social media profiles. And on that helpful but annoying sticky name tag at your next in-person event.

And ...

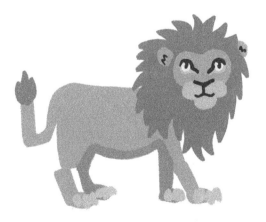

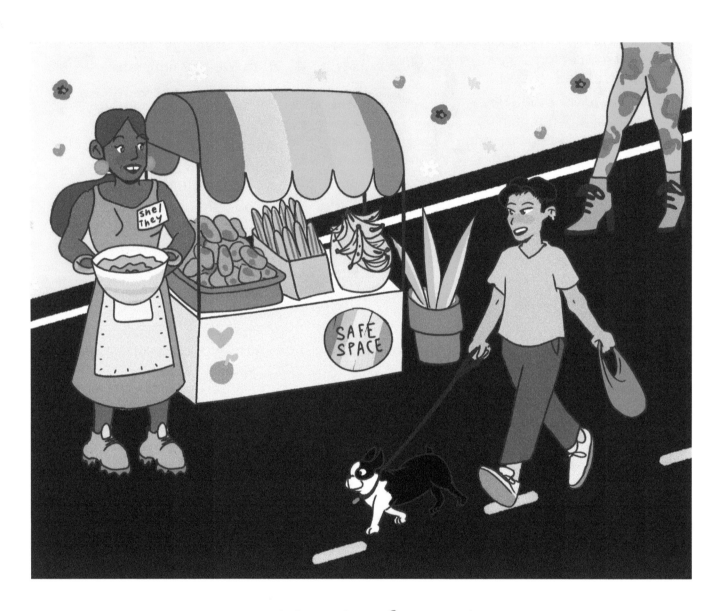

♥ Syd takes Winni for a walk. ♥

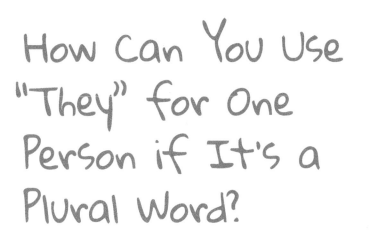

How Can You Use "They" for One Person if It's a Plural Word?

20

While I write this I'm waiting for the plumber to arrive, but I don't know exactly what time they'll be here.

Last week someone dropped their Whataburger™ wrapper on my driveway, and I had to put it into the trash for them.

I came home from a short trip last month and figured it must've stormed really badly while I was gone, as someone had left their business flyer on my slightly hail-damaged car.

Later this week I'm dog-sitting for my friend Thea (she/her), who has an adorable Boston Terrier called Winni. Thea hires a daily dog-walker, and she tells me that they love Winni even more than she does!

Get my point?

We actually have been using the word "they" in a singular meaning for centuries; it's just now that some people are realizing that they don't identify with being totally masculine or totally feminine that some other people have gotten into a little tizzy about it.

But guess what? There's even more history around this word than we might imagine. For hundreds and hundreds of years, people used they/them in the singular. Just one example from Shakespeare's *A Comedy of Errors* (1594), Act IV, Scene 3 reads:

> *There's not a man I meet but doth salute me*
> *As if I were their well-acquainted friend*

But then grammar gurus in the 18th century stepped in and decided that everyone should just use the male pronouns of "he" and "him" for all,[1] because it would be just much easier on everyone that way. I mean, it's not like they could've predicted how ridiculous something like "Every player on the women's soccer team thanked his family and wife," would sound, now is it?

I also find it curious that this was prevalent at a time when Queen Victoria (she/her), a woman, reigned over the British Empire, including many colonies. I guess those guys really wanted to control the masses, but I digress.

What's different this time is that more and more people are coming to realize that gender is a combination of a social construct and a human trait wired into our brains. While it was wrong that half the population had to agree to using male-only pronouns to keep the boys happy all those centuries ago, we now understand that just two gender pronouns are limiting too.

Gender is a spectrum with hundreds of real human experiences. Just because "male" and "female" are the two most commonly known, it doesn't mean the others don't exist. Think of a common fruit or vegetable and ask yourself if there are only two variations. For the life of me I've yet to come up with one. Even freaking potatoes have 4,000 varieties![2]

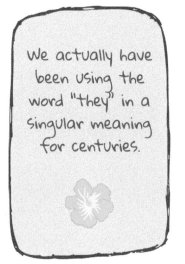

We actually have been using the word "they" in a singular meaning for centuries.

But using a person's correct pronouns can easily be a life or death situation, and I'm not exaggerating.

Trigger warning: According to the Trevor Project's *National Survey on LGBTQ Youth Mental Health 2021*, "42 percent of LGBTQ youth seriously considered attempting suicide in the past year, including more than half of transgender and nonbinary youth."[3]

If you are a young person considering suicide, please call the TrevorLifeline at 1-866-488-7386 or text "START" to 678-678 right now.

If you are over twenty-five years old and considering suicide, please call the National Suicide Prevention Lifeline at 1-800-273-8255 or text 988 right now.

Everyone else, think about it ... if someone used a wrong pronoun for you, how would you react? I can think of some straight, cis, male friends of mine who would be appalled if someone called them a girl. But those guys can brush it off and laugh if they choose, whereas for trans* and gender nonbinary people who are living in a world that typically only provides two options, it can be a daily struggle to exist. They simply don't belong in either of those buckets.

As our minds are wired to make assumptions about people based on how they look and sound *to us*, it's easy to accidentally make a mistake. Implicit—or unaware—thoughts make us choose pronouns for someone without even thinking. But pronouns are not a choice; they're an identity, and if we can catch ourselves before we make a guess, we can make someone's day.

No matter what someone looks or sounds like, I can say,

"Hi! My name's Fiona. I realize we can't tell by looking or how I sound, so know that my pronouns are she/her. May I know your name and pronouns too, please?"

If their reply is they/them, I use they/them. If he/him, I use he/him. If she/her, I use she/her. I'll use whichever pronouns someone tells me regardless of how they look or sound. And I encourage you to as well. Not only is using someone's correct pronouns respectful, the right words make people feel safe, seen, and validated.

And even better, as stated above, it can literally save their life.

If you want to get super supportive, participate each year on the third Wednesday of October when we honor International Pronouns Day. This commemoration was founded by Shige Sakurai (they/them), who also created the website mypronouns.org. There you can find free resources and educational pointers on how to apply pronouns correctly for all.

So it's not that hard, is it? Now lemme go answer the door as I see the plumber has just parked their vehicle outside.

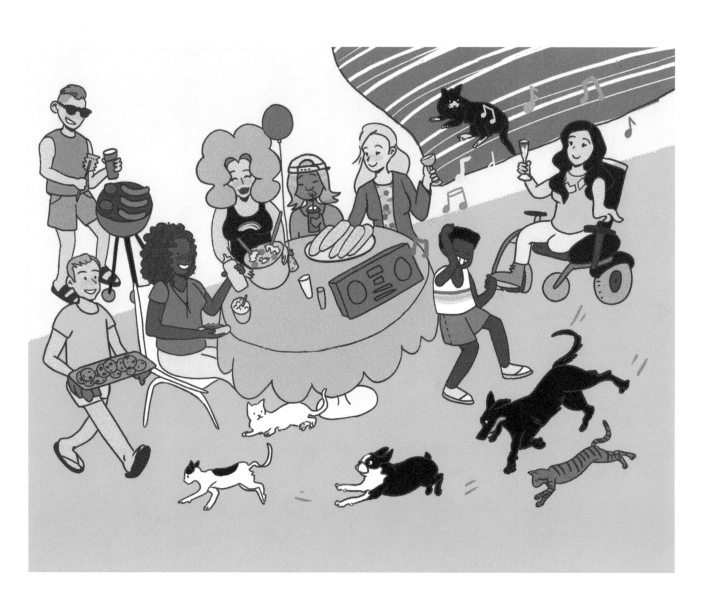

♥ Some of Fiona's closest family and friends—
and their fur-kids—having a cracking cookout! ♥

How Can I Keep My Kids Safe from Transgender and Gay People?

21

I used to work at the Houston Area Women's Center, which is a nonprofit organization helping survivors of domestic and sexual violence. It was there I learned that the highest risk of assault for any individual comes from the person they see in the mirror. Not ourselves, although arguably our own minds can beat us up from time to time, but the people we live with. Parents, spouses, siblings, significant others, and so on.

In other words, it's certainly not the creepy stranger we see depicted in films, television, and on the news. And it's definitely not transgender and gay people. As someone who has experienced sexual assault and domestic abuse, I can say in my personal experience that this rings true.

The Rape Abuse and Incest National Network reports that "As many as 93 percent of victims under the age of 18 know the abuser."[1] Let me be abundantly clear: children are more likely to be abused by someone they know than by a stranger.

It seems probable that cisgender and straight adults are just as likely to be abusers as transgender and gay people. Whereas studies show that transgender and gay adults are almost four times more likely to be victims of violent crime,[2] and LGBTQ+ children are at increased risk of child abuse, given only one in three young people live in LGBTQ affirming homes.[3]

What LGBTQIA+ and non-LGBTQIA+ people have in common is that the perpetrators are more likely to be someone they know.

Unfortunately, media has presented a biased portrayal of LGBTQIA+ people as "villains," or worse, "child molestors." You've gotta watch the ground-breaking documentary *Disclosure* to have your mind blown when you realize how centuries of pop-culture have warped our understanding of gender.

I think people who don't have friends—or don't *know* that they have friends—who are lesbian, gay, bisexual, transgender, queer, or any other identity outside of straight and cis, understandably have this notion that anyone with a penis is a potential real and present threat. Thanks, *Silence of the Lambs*.

Some men say they want to make sure transgender women stay out of the locker room because they know that if *they* were in there, they'd be wanting to eye up, or try it on, with the girls.[4] Ewwwww! Now *that* is someone I wouldn't want any child to be around. Because for goodness' sake, trans* and gay people just want to be able to get on with their lives without getting beaten up and/or murdered. That's the actual top-line of the "gay agenda."

Let's remember: gender identity is something every human being has wired into our brains. It's who we know ourselves to be, how we present ourselves to the world, and how the world sees us. Sexual orientation is a combination of love, romance, and/or sexual attraction towards another person.

Abusers are something else entirely. Abusers can be anyone with any gender identity and/or sexual orientation. In my mind, what's actually a form of abuse is making LGBTQIA+ kids go through so-called "conversion therapy." The Trevor Project found that kids who endure this type of "therapy" are twice as likely to attempt suicide than those who don't.[5]

Dear friends, if you are a young person considering suicide, please call the

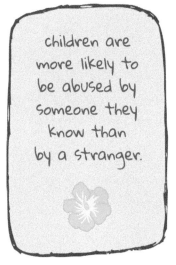

children are more likely to be abused by someone they know than by a stranger.

TrevorLifeline at 1-866-488-7386 or text "START" to 678-678 right now.

If you are over twenty-five years old and considering suicide, please call the National Suicide Prevention Lifeline at 1-800-273-8255 or text 988 right now.

Everyone else, let's get back to the question of how to keep your kids safe from transgender and gay people.

♥ **Step one:** realize that there's no danger to your children from transgender and gay, or any LGBTQIA+ person, simply because of their gender identity and/or sexual orientation.

♥ **Step two:** realize that actually building genuine friendships and letting your kids know people who are LGBTQIA+ creates community. And community is always a good thing.

♥ **Step three:** realize that including LGBTQIA+ people in your life could be saving your own kid's life. More and more young people are breaking the binary of gender and sexuality and coming out as LGBTQ+,[6] and they're more likely to harm themselves or be harmed if they don't feel safe being themselves at home.

Supportive families are vital to ensuring that kids are raised to be happy, healthy, and protected from discrimination.

♥ **Step four:** take action. There are many days throughout the year when we go out of our way to show love and appreciation for our fellow humans. Pick a recognition day and take the kids in your life to a charity event, a volunteer day, or even a Transgender Day of Remembrance vigil; although I'd highly recommend going out for ice-cream with the participants after, because damn, those candlelit ceremonies are seriously depressing.

Bottom line: be kind and courageous.

Peace, y'all.

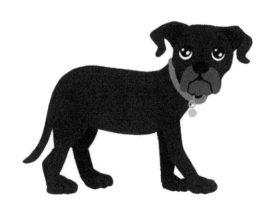

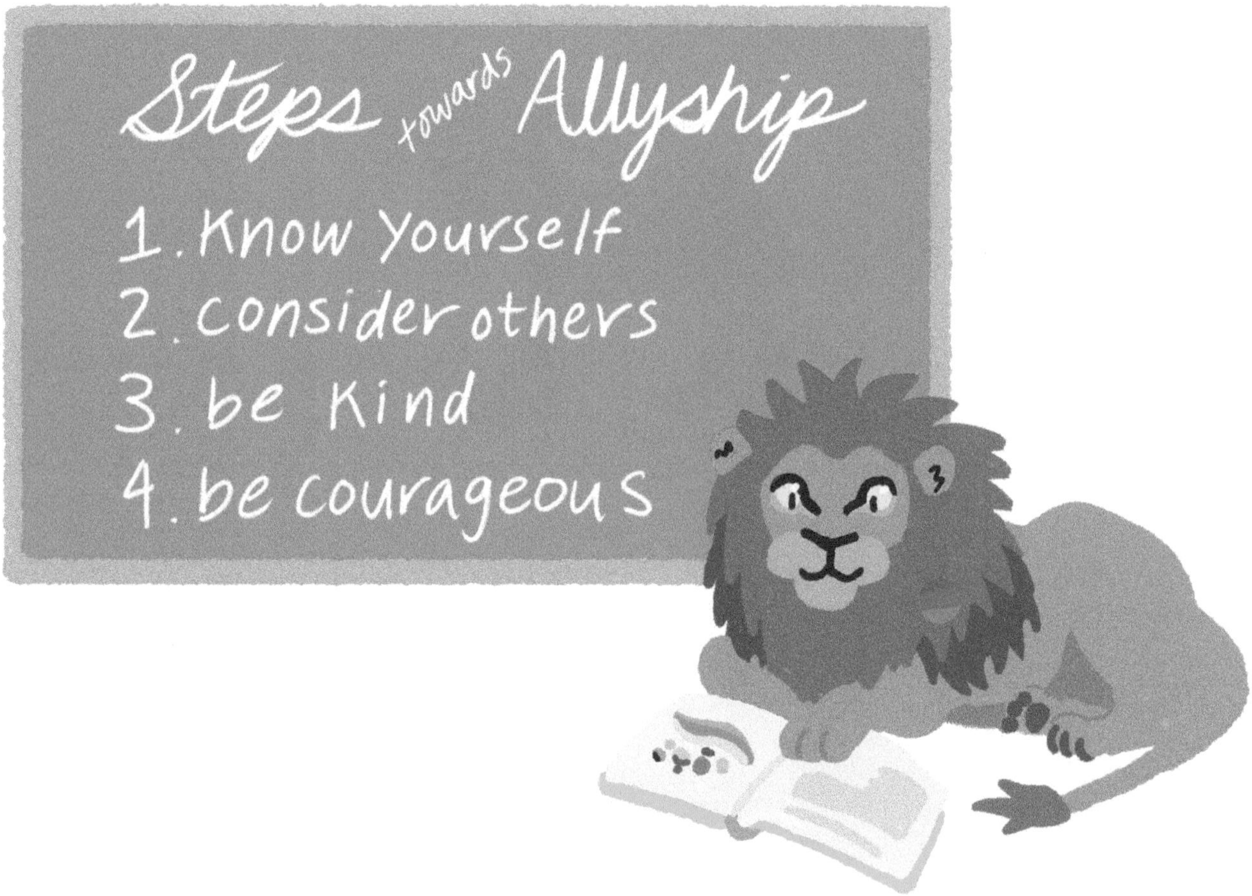
Steps towards Allyship
1. Know yourself
2. consider others
3. be kind
4. be courageous

Conclusion: How Can I Be the Best Ally Ever?!

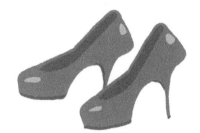

The simplest way I can describe how to be an ally is to be kind and courageous.

If you've read and digested all 21 chapters, then you're ready to put on your cape, click your heels, and get out into the world like a badass LGBTQIA+ crusader. However, we don't all need to take our action to the same degree.

Remember, everything in life is a spectrum, and we all have different roles to play. So don't judge yourself for what you do or don't do. Just don't be an asshole.

Seriously, if you want to be an ally and not an asshole, I'd suggest you take these four steps:

Step one: know yourself.

♥ Have the ability to describe easily and quickly what "cisgender" means. Either use the description in this book or share this link to my two-minute explainer video: bitly.com/CisTransExplainer to those who don't know.

♥ Consider how you yourself fall within, or outside, the spectrums of gender and sexual orientation.

My friends Hunter Rook (he/they), Jay Mays (she/they), and Robin Mack (they/name only), who created the brilliant thegenderbook.com, can help you figure it out.

♥ Remember that your biological sex is not the same as your gender. They might be related and help each other out a little, but your junk does not determine who you go to bed as, nor who you go to bed with.

♥ Don't ask people you don't know well about their private parts or how they have sex. When you get to know LGBTQIA+ people, check yourself on any curiosity to ask them about their genitals, the name they were given at birth (some people call this a "dead name"[1]), or other personal and medical history. And definitely get to know someone really well before you ask about their private life! Allow your new friend to have the space to be able to share as much or as little as they like. Live in the present and accept that person as they are today. Be mindful.

♥ Use your privilege. When our gender meets society's expectations, we experience an easier time in the world. Those of us who easily conform have an opportunity to speak up for those whose gender does not neatly fall into one of society's silly boxes.

Step two: consider others.

♥ Learn more about the spectrum of identities and share your knowledge with the world. Hell, gift this book or any of my recommended reading to everyone you know.

♥ Add in layers of knowledge around gender and sexuality identities within race and ethnicity considerations. Studies show that in the United States, non-white people are more likely to identify as LGBTQ+ than white people. This is because younger people are more likely to be out as LGBTQ+ than older people. And with changing US demographics, younger people are more likely to be non-white.[2] So when you are looking at issues of biased incarceration, employment, healthcare, etc. you come to realize that you can't exclude LGBTQIA+ people from other efforts to build equity.

♥ Listen. So many courageous people are sharing their stories in multiple ways online, on podcasts, on YouTube channels, in books, etc. We can learn from hearing other people's life experiences and oftentimes they help us navigate our own. Be mindful that you don't know what you don't know, but there's always the opportunity to gain knowledge through active listening.

♥ Be empathetic. When I was working on the feature documentary

TransMilitary, I didn't know what it felt like to be transgender (nor serve in the military for that matter), but I did know intimately how it feels to be seen as someone you're not. To varying degrees, practically all people understand feelings of anxiety, depression, fear, powerlessness, and being "othered." We can also relate to being respected, powerful, worthy, loved, and included. Even though our circumstances are different, we can empathize with other people's emotions and show kindness and courage in our actions.

Step three: be kind.

♥ Politely ask for someone's pronouns, and not their "preferred" pronouns. This isn't like asking for someone's wine preference, but if you're wondering I'll take red, please! As I indicated earlier, I typically say something like …

"Hi! My name's Fiona. I realize we can't tell by looking or how we sound, so know that my pronouns are she/her. May I know your name and pronouns too, please?"

Put your pronouns on video calls, email signatures, and introduce yourself with your pronouns at a meeting regardless of who's attending. We can never assume someone's identity by the way they look or sound, and these actions are ally pro tips. If someone questions why it's important, you can send them to mypronouns.org.

♥ If you're ever not sure about someone's pronouns and it's not the right time to ask, use their name until you know. Just do not make a guess. This is also a good practice when talking about someone's partner(s) as we shouldn't make assumptions about the gender(s) of who someone is in relationship(s) with.

♥ Practice patience with all people in your life. Being patient with a person who is questioning or exploring their gender identity and/or sexual orientation is extremely important. No human being is born with a manual, and it can take a while to figure ourselves out. Like straight and cisgender people, LGBTQIA+ people's paths to know and express themselves are unique and personal. There's no right or wrong way to self-discovery and expression, but there are definitely right ways to supportively affirm someone's experience. Period.

♥ Hey y'all, use gender-inclusive language, always. Even when you're with straight, cisgender people. Once you realize how we're perpetuating sexist language it's hard to unhear it. We've also been using gender-neutral language our entire lives too. You think all lives matter? Then use all-inclusive language.

♥ Give time, talent, and/or treasure to nonprofit organizations that help advance LGBTQIA+ equality. You can find a list of suggestions at the back of this book.

Step four: be courageous.

♥ Speak up. I know I'm repeating this one, but seriously, silence can be complicity. Being a badass LGBTQIA+ ally is rooted in using your voice in whichever form suits you best to not only call out

violence and discrimination, but to help educate those who don't understand and are fearful of difference. Whether it be sharing films, books, or viral TikToks with loved ones, having a heavy offline conversation, or backing someone up in public, being an upstander is critical for human equity. The rights of a minority were never won without the support of the majority.

♥ When you mess up, say you're sorry and move on. I say "when," because even the best-intentioned of us mess up, but don't rub salt into the wound by making your mess-up the focus of the conversation. The LGBTQIA+ person you're talking with doesn't need an explanation of how hard you're trying, or how difficult it is for you to use their name. They just need you to keep doing your best as practice makes perfect.

♥ Create a platform and recognize when to take a seat. Not all LGBTQIA+ people want to explain or educate the world about their lives and bodies. But some LGBTQIA+ people do. Finding a balance between being a vocal advocate but not taking the stage when an LGBTQIA+ person should be up there is a call back to our own self-awareness. Form genuine friendships with a variety of people in your life and live with a mindset of abundance rather than lack. When you see an opportunity for an LGBTQIA+ person to have a job they love or be seen and heard on a platform they aspire to, make introductions and step out of the way.

♥ Before you vote for a political candidate, learn their stated positions on LGBTQIA+ issues. Then vote with your intentions to be an ally in mind.

♥ Empower people, including politicians, who genuinely want to provide equitable provisions for life, liberty, and the pursuit of happiness for all.

LGBTQIA+ people have existed for as long as humanity has existed. The time to increase our consciousness and decolonize our worldview of gender and sexuality for our collective greater good is right now.

Bottom line: don't be an asshole. Be kind and courageous.

Thank you.

Acknowledgments

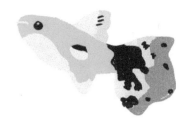

I swear writing the acknowledgments page is harder than writing the damn book! Every single person who's ever touched my life in any way is due some appreciation for inspiring me to create *What Does That LGBTQIA+ Label Mean?* And I bet there are a ton of people I've never even met that have somehow sent magic my way through the Universe. So in essence please know that I ooze love and gratitude for you all, including you my dear reader, whether your name is mentioned here or not.

Firstly, thank you to Jenn T. Grace for empowering people like me to share our stories with the world. Your last name reflects how you are living your mission. I know firsthand that you deliver your smarts and determination with reassuring calm and grace. Jenn, you and your Publish Your Purpose team are a joy to collaborate with and I'm grateful for our friendship that has blossomed through our working relationship. Thank you Bailly Morse for your always on-the-ball and responsive management, and your edit. Thank you Niki Garcia for seamlessly streaming the workflow behind my scenes, August Li for your mindful developmental edit, Lisa Canfield for your insightful copy edit, Lori McFerran for your meticulous and enlightening proofread, and Nelly Murariu for designing the book with graphics and

Syd's illustrations to look so freaking gorgeous.

Also thank you, thank you, to my friend and über talented Creative Director, Marc Nahas, who has donated so much of his time and talent for my *NOW with Fiona* and Free Lion Productions logos, brand, motion graphics, and other marvelous elements.

Thank you Kristina Marusic, Syd Cordoba, August Li, Trish King, Lilith Kidd, Daley South and Dixie Krystals for giving thumbs up on my explanations, especially when I have not experienced all of their identities.

The day New York City shut down due to the pandemic in March 2020, I was sitting in a lovely lunch spot in Lake Jackson, Texas with one of my besties, Julz. For various reasons, panic shot through my body and my gut screamed that I needed to move out of Brooklyn, ASAP. Without skipping a beat Julz said, "Come live with me. For as long as you want," and she meant it. Literally. So I flew back the next day, threw essentials into my car, and drove over 1,700 miles from NYC to Julz's home in south-central Brazoria County. I thought I'd be there until May and then move to Austin, lmao. I ended up staying with her and her sons for just under ten months. For Julz, Jake, Max, and Julz's partner Roy, I have endless gratitude. You saved my ass, but the bonus was that going from Brooklyn to B'County made many rich memories with new and glorious friends like the Lezak family, Rochelle, and John. And my sweet little deplorable, Zane. I couldn't have planned for the insightful fodder that emerged from that small Texas town for this book and the next.

When the feature documentary *TransMilitary*, which I made with my dear friends and talented co-creators Gabe Silverman and Jamie Coughlin premiered at SXSW 2018, I had no idea that a chance meeting at that festival with Sheila Grace Newsome would lead me to the extraordinary Mindy Raymond. I'm first dibs in claiming Mindy as The Media Mogul of Texas. I'm indebted for her and Sheila's faith, tenacity, and loyalty towards our shared dreams and goals, especially with *NOW with Fiona*. I'm delighted that Mindy and her husband Nate, and their kiddos Jack and Andrew, and Mindy's Momma Linda have become my new family-I-choose.

Speaking of family-you-choose, here's a list of heartfelt mentions ... Dwayne Beebe and Sean Martin, Brittany Burch, Vance Nesbitt and Jeff Havard, Katherine Willis and Charlie, Amanda Plocheck, Chris McNeany and Tom Lavoie, Logan and Laila Ireland, my entire *TransMilitary* family, Rhys Harper, Ryan Levy and Ian Eastveld, Amanda Simpson and Jennifer Watkins, Brian, George, Arya, Gaia and Gareth O'Leary-Appling, Karen Campbell, Ashley Nichols and Pete Bailey, Jonathan Franqui, John Becker, Emil Pagliarulo, David Newton, Greg and Beth Brown, Heather Page and Todd McMullen, Sheri Swokowski, Ariel Lopez and Josh Becker, and Tim Berry. It was Tim, btw, who after listening to my intentions with the book said to me, "Oh! So basically you're working to decolonize gender and sexuality." I excitedly jumped out of my seat exclaiming, "Yes! Wow! I didn't know that saying was actually a thing!"

I'm grateful for the friendship and camaraderie I share with Brynn Tannehill, who opened my world to transgender service members in 2012 and still today she remains a go-to for facts and figures—including quantifying private parts surgeries for this book. And thank goodness for Allyson Robinson, who years ago first taught me about the foundations of breaking down gender, as her presentation set me off on this whole journey. Around the same time, Landon Marchant was the first transgender service member I interviewed on camera and their vulnerability, openness, and trust in me helped build a solid foundation for my own education. Thank you my dear Landon. You are another chosen sibling.

Thank you Kristina Marusic for keeping me in the know on #Bisexual TikTok, Crystal Nuding for keeping me chill with conscious creation business coaching, and Robin Mack for keeping me confident with smarts on all things gender. When it comes to mindfulness and helping me dig through my shit, I give praise and gratitude for Angela Mendes. Thank you Dawn Ennis for our friendship and being a trusted fact finder, and Joanna Harper for also endeavoring to track factual resources.

Thank you to Syd Cordoba for the talent and collaboration you brought to the manuscript and illustrations featuring themself, several of our friends and family, and Kate Sephora Del Castillo, Laila and Logan Ireland, Jessica Ping-Wild, Daley South, Dixie Krystals, Raffi Freedman-Gurspan, Edie Windsor,

Fred Martinez, Jr., Neneh Diallo, Jayde McFarlane and Tyler Lyons, Monica Roberts, Chris McNeany, the cats Princess Piggy, Lazy Boy, Teeshka, and Pepito. Gus, Sooty, Tess, Ponce, and Cheese didn't make the final cut, but we did manage to squeeze in the dogs Hondo and Winni, and the pitbull-boxer mix love of my life, Ms. Maizie Rai.

Which brings me to the family in which I was born, who are probably wondering what the hell happened during my upbringing. I know Dad actually wonders how on earth he and my mum produced me, lol. I put some of it down to the love and kinship we shared within our family circle of which my mother, Jane, was the driving force. Mummy died in 2006 at the age of 54 from pancreatic cancer, but I know that she's with us in Spirit every single day. I give gratitude for the open and loving mindset she fostered and how she brought us all together with her sisters Aunty Susie, Aunty Sarah, and Aunty Clare. You might be able to tell from Chapter One that Clare and I have a unique bond that holds us together no matter the time and distance between. Thank you Clare for helping me in ways most people don't know.

The love and kinship continue with my cousins Sam, Tom, Matthew, Nick, and Emma, although my Emma is more like a younger sister and she happens to be hilarious. Emma used to tell me when she was ten and I was 13 that she thought I was a lesbian and, although I didn't know it at the time, she wasn't far off.

I give thanks and love for one of the funniest people I know, my brother Rob and his beautifully soulful wife, Jessica. Their quiet confidence inspires me to consciously create the life I envision, just as they are living theirs. And I totally wish I could steal their dog, Tara and pet their cat Zulu more often.

I'm grateful my sister has the love and affection of the beautiful family she's created, starting with her number one constant teammate for the last 14 years, her son, Oscar. Today, with her husband, Chris, and step-daughters, Ella and Talie, they complete their happy unit with my dear nephew. Oscar is the apple of my eye who I want to grow up to live in a world that doesn't box any human into silly rules and expectations. Oscar is a witty and kind person; a proud reflection of his dad Paul, Step-Mum Lu, and his mum; my incredible sister, Joanna aka Lilibet.

There's no other woman alive on this planet who I can feel more love for than my Lilibet. Being her Margot is my greatest blessing. If the dedication to Dad in my first book hadn't been so funny then she would've been there in the beginning. So Joey, my Lilibet, I'm delighted I had to quickly get this "safe-for-work" version out and could dedicate it to you. There's no greater champion I have in life than you, although Clare would give you a run for your money! Joey, you are the epitome of kindness and courage.

Finally, dear Jenny and Dad. I'm so happy and grateful that you have each other to share life, love, and laughs together. Thank you for all the ways you both show and give roots to our sprawling family. It's also a blessing that I don't have to plan on returning to the UK to wipe Dad's arse when he's too old, so thanks for that as well, Jenny ;). And Dad, thank you so much for raising me to be a daughter that, in your presence, can confidently tell you anything. Literally anything. I love you.

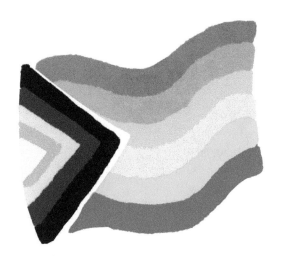

ADDITIONAL RESOURCES

YOUTUBE VIDEOS

♥ Fiona's Coming Out as Bisexual Video (a bit outdated but still relevant): bitly.com/bifiona

♥ Intersexion: Boy or Girl? (Intersex Documentary) | Real Stories: https://youtu.be/czbQRjdGvYQ

♥ Pidgeon: Intersex Stories (Not Surgeries): youtube.com/user/pidgejen

♥ Two-minute animated explainer on the difference between "cisgender" and "transgender" (hire me to make more videos like this for your company or organization): bitly.com/CisTransExplainer

FILMS

♥ Changing the Game: https://www.imdb.com/title/tt10011320/

♥ Disclosure: https://www.imdb.com/title/tt8637504/

♥ For the Bible Tells Me So: https://www.imdb.com/title/tt0912583/

♥ 1946: The Mistranslation That Shifted a Culture: https://www.imdb.com/title/tt10389180/

♥ More Than He Knows: https://www.imdb.com/title/tt8869814/

♥ My Octopus Teacher: https://www.imdb.com/title/tt12888462/

♥ Pray Away: https://www.imdb.com/title/tt11224358/

♥ TransMilitary: transmilitary.org

♥ Transgender, at War and in Love: bitly.com/loganandlaila

BOOKS

♥ Boylan, Jennifer Finney. She's Not There: A Life in Two Genders. New York: Crown Publishing Group, 2003

♥ Grace, m.d., Sheila. A Calling from the Bones. Austin: Sheila Rising Books, 2018

♥ Stryker, Susan. Transgender History: The Roots of Today's Revolution. New York: Seal Press, 2017

♥ Tolle, Eckhart. The Power of Now: A Guide to Spiritual Enlightenment. California: New World Library, 2004

♥ Vaid-Menon, Alok. Beyond the Gender Binary. New York: Penguin Random House, 2020

♥ Zaki, Jamil. The War for Kindness: Building Empathy in a Fractured World. New York: Crown, 2019

♥ Mack, Robin, Mays, Jay, and Rook, Hunter. The Gender Book. Houston: Publisher Marshall House Press, 2014

PODCASTS

♥ LGBTQ&A hosted by Jeffrey Masters / The Advocate magazine in partnership with GLAAD

♥ The Laverne Cox Show hosted by Laverne Cox

♥ The Will to Change: Uncovering True Stories of Diversity & Inclusion hosted by Jennifer Brown

MORE LGBTQIA+ LANGUAGE THINGS TO KNOW

- ♥ LGBTQIA Wiki: lgbtqia.fandom.com
- ♥ PFLAG National Glossary of Terms: pflag.org/glossary
- ♥ Pronouns Matter: mypronouns.org
- ♥ The Gender Book: thegenderbook.com

ORGANIZATIONS TO SUPPORT AND LEARN FROM

If you are a young person considering suicide, please call the TrevorLifeline at 1-866-488-7386 right now.

If you are over twenty-five years old and considering suicide, please call the National Suicide Prevention Lifeline at 1-800-273-8255 right now.

BISEXUAL

- ♥ Bisexual.org: bi.org
- ♥ Bisexual Resource Center: biresource.org

FAMILIES, inc. YOUTH and AGEING

- ♥ interACT: Advocates for Intersex Youth: interactadvocates.org
- ♥ PFLAG: pflag.org
- ♥ Services and Advocacy for Gay, Lesbian, Bisexual & Transgender Elders (SAGE): sageusa.org
- ♥ The Trevor Project: thetrevorproject.org

GENERAL

- ♥ American Institute of Bisexuality: americaninstituteofbisexuality.org
- ♥ Human Rights Campaign Foundation: hrc.org or thehrcfoundation.org
- ♥ Matthew Shepard Foundation: matthewshepard.org

- ♥ Movement Advancement Project: lgbtmap.org
- ♥ Straight for Equality (outreach and education by PFLAG): straightforequality.org
- ♥ Two Spirit Nation: thetwospiritnation.org

LEGAL

- ♥ American Civil Liberties Union (ACLU): aclu.org
- ♥ Lambda Legal: lambdalegal.org
- ♥ National Center for Lesbian Rights: nclrights.org
- ♥ The Sylvia Rivera Law Project: srlp.org
- ♥ Transgender Legal Defense & Education Fund: transgenderlegal.org
- ♥ Transgender Law Center: transgenderlawcenter.org

MEDIA

- ♥ GLAAD: glaad.org
- ♥ NLGJA: The Association of LGBTQ Journalists: nlgja.org

MILITARY

- ♥ Modern Military Association of America: modernmilitary.org
- ♥ Palm Center: palmcenter.org
- ♥ SPARTA: spartapride.org

POLITICAL and/or LEGAL

- ♥ Equality Federation: equalityfederation.org
- ♥ Equality Texas: equalitytexas.org
- ♥ GLBTQ Legal Advocates & Defenders (GLAD): glad.org
- ♥ Human Rights Campaign: hrc.org
- ♥ Immigration Equality: immigrationequality.org

- ♥ National Center for Transgender Equality: transequality.org
- ♥ National LGBTQ Task Force: thetaskforce.org
- ♥ Victory Fund: victoryfund.org

SCHOOL

- ♥ GLSEN: glsen.org
- ♥ Point Foundation: pointfoundation.org
- ♥ Welcoming Schools: welcomingschools.org

SPORTS

- ♥ Athlete Ally: athleteally.org
- ♥ Changing the Game: changinggamedoc.com

WORK

- ♥ Out & Equal Workplace Advocates: outandequal.org

FIND DIXIE KRYSTALS AND DRAG QUEEN STORYTIME

- ♥ dixiekrystals.com

BIBLIOGRAPHY

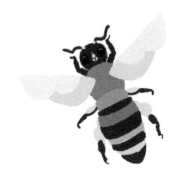

Quote

1. Vaid-Menon, Alok. *Beyond the Gender Binary*. Penguin Workshop, 2020. Accessed: June 4, 2021. https://www.goodreads.com/author/quotes/19436850.Alok_Vaid_Menon

Introduction

1. Cahalan, Rose. "TransMilitary' Is the LGBT Advocacy Film Middle America Needs to See." *The Texas Observer. Accessed: June 4, 2021.* https://www.texasobserver.org/transmilitary-is-the-lgbt-advocacy-film-middle-america-needs-to-see/

2. Mallory, Christy, Taylor N.T. Brown, Stephen Russell & Brad Sears. "The Impact of Stigma and Discrimination Against LGBT People in Texas." The Williams Institute. Accessed: June 4, 2021. https://williamsinstitute.law.ucla.edu/wp-content/uploads/Impact-LGBT-Discrimination-TX-Apr-2017.pdf

What's the Difference between "Cisgender" and "Transgender?"

1. Nguyen HB, Loughead J, Lipner E, Hantsoo L, Kornfield SL, Epperson CN. "What has sex got to do with it? The role of hormones in the transgender brain." Neuropsychopharmacology: official publication of the American College of Neuropsychopharmacology vol. 44,1 (2019): 22-37. https://www.ncbi.nlm.nih.gov/pmc/articles/PMC6235900/

What Does It Mean to Be Intersex?

1. Blackless, Melanie, Anthony Charuvastra, Amanda Derryck, Anne Fausto-Sterling, Karl Lauzanne, and Ellen Lee. "How sexually dimorphic are we? Review and synthesis." *American Journal of Human Biology 12:151-166.* https://pubmed.ncbi.nlm.nih.gov/11534012/

2. interACT: Advocates for Intersex Youth. "FAQ: What is intersex?" interACT. Accessed: June 4, 2021. https://interactadvocates.org/faq/

3. Cunningham A L, Jones C P, Ansell J, Barry J D. "Red for danger: the effects of red hair in surgical practice." *BMJ 2010 341.* https://www.bmj.com/content/341/bmj.c6931

4. interACT: Advocates for Intersex Youth. "FAQ: What is intersex?" interACT. Accessed: June 4, 2021. https://interactadvocates.org/faq/

Do Transgender Men Actually Exist?

1. Human Rights Campaign Foundation. "An Epidemic of Violence: Fatal Violence Against Transgender and Gender Nonconforming People in The United States In 2020." The Human Rights Campaign. Accessed: June 4, 2021. https://hrc-prod-requests.s3-us-west-2.amazonaws.com/FatalViolence-2020Report-Final.pdf?mtime=20201119101455&focal=none

2. Meyer, Ilan H., Bianca D.M. Wilson, and Kathryn O'Neill. "LGBTQ People in the US: Select Findings from the Generations and TransPop Studies." The Williams Institute. Accessed: June 4, 2021. https://williamsinstitute.law.ucla.edu/publications/generations-transpop-toplines/

3. Mekelburg, Madlin. "Fact-check: What does the law say about children and sex reassignment surgery?" *Austin American-Statesman. Accessed: June 4, 2021.* https://www.statesman.com/news/20191111/fact-check-what-does-law-say-about-children-and-sex-reassignment-surgery

4. The Trevor Project. "National Survey on LGBTQ Youth Mental Health 2021." The Trevor Project. Accessed: June 4, 2021. https://www.thetrevorproject.org/survey-2021

5. Growing Up Transgender. "Puberty Blockers – Overview of the research." Accessed: June 4, 2021. https://growinguptransgender.com/2020/06/10/puberty-blockers-overview-of-the-research/

6. Wilson, Lena. "What Are Puberty Blockers?" *The New York Times. Accessed: June 4, 2021.* https://www.nytimes.com/2021/05/11/well/family/what-are-puberty-blockers.html

7. Growing Up Transgender. "Puberty Blockers – Overview of the research." Accessed: June 4, 2021. https://growinguptransgender.com/2020/06/10/puberty-blockers-overview-of-the-research/

Is Being Nonbinary Just Cool These Days?

1. Wilson, Bianca D.M., and Ilan H. Meyer. "Nonbinary LGBTQ Adults in the United States." The Williams Institute. Accessed: June 4, 2021. https://williamsinstitute.law.ucla.edu/publications/nonbinary-lgbtq-adults-us/

2. Burling, Robbins. *The strong women of Modhupur. Dhaka: The University Press Limited, 1997.*

3. Gettleman, Jeffrey. *"The Peculiar Position of India's Third Gender."* The New York Times. Accessed: June 4, 2021. https://www.nytimes.com/2018/02/17/style/india-third-gender-hijras-transgender.html

4. The Human Rights Campaign Foundation. "Seven Things About Transgender People That You Didn't Know." The Human Rights Campaign. Accessed: June 4, 2021. https://www.hrc.org/resources/seven-things-about-transgender-people-that-you-didnt-know

5. National Park Foundation Washington, DC. "LGBTQ America: A Theme Study of Lesbian, Gay, Bisexual, Transgender, and Queer History." National Park Foundation and the National Park Service. Accessed: June 4, 2021. https://www.nps.gov/subjects/lgbtqheritage/upload/lgbtqtheme-nativeamerica.pdf

6. The National Archives. "What was early contact like between English colonists and Native Americans?" The National Archives. Accessed: June 4, 2021. https://www.nationalarchives.gov.uk/education/resources/native-north-americans/

Are Drag Queens Transgender?

1. Abrams, Mere. "64 Terms That Describe Gender Identity and Expression." Healthline. Accessed: June 4, 2021. https://www.healthline.com/health/different-genders

Are Bisexuals Just Greedy?

1. Gates, Gary J. "How Many People are Lesbian, Gay, Bisexual, and Transgender?" The Williams Institute. Accessed: July 4, 2021. https://williamsinstitute.law.ucla.edu/publications/how-many-people-lgbt/

Which One Is Better, Bisexual or Pansexual?

1. Gates, Gary J. "How Many People are Lesbian, Gay, Bisexual, and Transgender?" The Williams Institute. Accessed: July 4, 2021. https://williamsinstitute.law.ucla.edu/publications/how-many-people-lgbt/

2. Mattison, Lindsay D. "Here's Every Type of Cherry and How to Use It." Taste of Home. Accessed: June 4, 2021. https://www.tasteofhome.com/collection/types-of-cherries/#:~:text=Although%20they're%20often%20simply,store%20cherries%20like%20a%20pro

Why Are We Saying, "Hey Guys!" to Greet Women?

1. YouTube Culture & Trends. "How do you welcome your fans to the show?" YouTube. Accessed: June 4, 2021. https://www.youtube.com/trends/articles/hey-guys/

2. History.com. "The death of Guy Fawkes." History. Accessed July 4, 2021. https://www.history.com/this-day-in-history/the-death-of-guy-fawkes

3. Greenspan, Jesse. "Guy Fawkes Day: A Brief History." History. Accessed: June 4, 2021. https://www.history.com/news/guy-fawkes-day-a-brief-history

4. Dewey, Caitlin. "An unnecessarily long and surprisingly fascinating history of 'guys'." *The Washington Post. Accessed: June 4, 2021.* https://www.washingtonpost.com/news/the-intersect/wp/2014/10/24/an-unnecessarily-long-and-surprisingly-fascinating-history-of-guys/?noredirect=on

Do All Transgender Men Want Male Genitalia?

1. Kime, Patricia. "DoD spends $84M a year on Viagra, similar meds." *Military Times. Accessed: July 4, 2021.* https://www.militarytimes.com/pay-benefits/military-benefits/health-care/2015/02/13/dod-spends-84m-a-year-on-viagra-similar-meds/

2. Janak, Judson C., Jean A. Orman, Douglas W. Soderdahl, and Steven J. Hudak. "Epidemiology of Genitourinary Injuries among Male US Service Members Deployed to Iraq and Afghanistan: Early Findings from the Trauma Outcomes and Urogenital Health (TOUGH) Project." *Journal of Urology. Accessed: July 7, 2021.* https://www.auajournals.org/doi/10.1016/j.juro.2016.08.005

3. Arnett, George. "Germany: the world's capital of penis enlargement." *The Guardian. Accessed: July 7, 2021.* https://www.theguardian.com/news/datablog/2014/jul/31/germany-the-worlds-capital-of-penis-enlargment-country

4. International Society of Aesthetic Plastic Surgery. "Why penile procedures are becoming so popular." International Society of Aesthetic Plastic Surgery. Accessed: July 7, 2021. https://www.isaps.org/blog/penile-procedures-becoming-popular/

5. Nolan, Ian T., Christopher J. Kuhner, and Geolani W. Dy. "Demographic and temporal trends in transgender identities and gender confirming surgery." *Translational Andrology and Urology vol. 8: 184-190.* https://www.ncbi.nlm.nih.gov/pmc/articles/PMC6626314/

How Do Transgender Women Pee in a Public Restroom?

1. Maza, Carlos. "Debunking The Big Myth About Transgender-Inclusive Bathrooms." Media Matters for America. Accessed: July 4, 2021. https://www.mediamatters.org/fox-nation/debunking-big-myth-about-transgender-inclusive-bathrooms

2. Flores, Andrew R., Ilan H. Meyer, Lynn Langton, and Jody L. Herman. "Gender Identity Disparities in Criminal Victimization." The Williams Institute. Accessed: July 4, 2021. https://williamsinstitute.law.ucla.edu/publications/ncvs-trans-victimization/

Why Does Allowing Athletes who are Transgender to Compete in School Sports Make America Great?

1. Rummler, Orion. "Which states have banned trans youth in sports." Axios. Accessed: July 4, 2021. https://www.axios.com/trans-youth-sports-ban-75e1c476-1ee7-42ea-9292-2f3bcce5d4d0.html

2. Goldberg, Shoshana K. "Fair Play. The Importance of Sports Participation for Transgender Youth." Center for American Progress. Accessed: June 4, 2021. https://www.americanprogress.org/issues/lgbtq-rights/reports/2021/02/08/495502/fair-play/

3. IOC Medical Commission Chairman Ljungqvist, Arne. "IOC approves consensus with regard to athletes who have changed sex." International Olympic Committee. Accessed: June 4, 2021. https://olympics.com/ioc/news/ioc-approves-consensus-with-regard-to-athletes-who-have-changed-sex-1

4. The Associated Press. "First openly transgender Olympians are competing in Tokyo." NBC Out News. Accessed: August 11, 2021. https://www.nbcnews.com/nbc-out/out-news/first-openly-transgender-olympians-are-competing-tokyo-rcna1507

5. Clymer, Charlotte. "Trans Panic and the Courage of Laurel Hubbard." Charlotte's Web Thoughts. Accessed: August 11, 2021. https://charlotteclymer.substack.com/p/trans-panic-and-the-courage-of-laurel-7df?justPublished=true

6. Blackless, Melanie, Anthony Charuvastra, Amanda Derryck, Anne Fausto-Sterling, Karl Lauzanne, and Ellen Lee. "How sexually dimorphic are we? Review and synthesis." *American Journal of Human Biology 12:151-166.* https://pubmed.ncbi.nlm.nih.gov/11534012/

7. Bollinger, Alex. "This video destroys Republican support for transgender sports bans." LGBTQ Nation. Accessed: July 4, 2021. https://www.lgbtqnation.com/2021/03/video-destroys-republican-support-transgender-sports-bans/?utm_

source=LGBTQ+Nation+Subscribers&utm_campaign=16f2a76404-20210326_LGBTQ_Nation_Daily_Brief&utm_medium=email&utm_term=0_c4eab596bd-16f2a76404-429797001

8. Strangio, Chase, and Gabriel Arkles. "Four Myths About Trans Athletes, Debunked." American Civil Liberties Union. Accessed: June 4, 2021. https://www.aclu.org/news/lgbt-rights/four-myths-about-trans-athletes-debunked/

9. Aspen Institute. "The Aspen Institute's Project Play explores the state of youth sports in 2020." Aspen Institute. Accessed: June 4, 2021. https://www.aspenprojectplay.org/state-of-play-2020/ages-6-12

10. Burns, Katelyn. "The massive Republican push to ban trans athletes, explained." Vox. Accessed: July 4, 2021. https://www.vox.com/identities/22334014/trans-athletes-bills-explained

11. Stahl, Shane. "Mythbuster: Debunking Anti-Transgender Messages." Freedom For All Americans. Accessed: July 4, 2021. https://freedomforallamericans.org/mythbuster-debunking-anti-transgender-messages/?gclid=CjwKCAjwulWHBhBDEiwACXQYseFrsWFiLUEuLT4mD9T_pM4FiVaewrM1jebOtdGvPAo7HDoSGT36IBoC5UAQAvD_BwE

12. Cox, Matthew. "Army Leaders Say ACFT 3.0 Remains Gender-Neutral, Despite Gender-Specific Evaluation Categories." Military.com. Accessed: July 4, 2021. https://www.military.com/daily-news/2021/03/22/army-leaders-say-acft-30-remains-gender-neutral-despite-gender-specific-evaluation-categories.html

Why Can't I Love the Sinner but Hate the Sin?

1. Mycio, Mary. "Archeology Isn't for Prudes." Slate. Accessed: June 4, 2021. https://slate.com/technology/2013/02/prehistoric-pornography-chinese-carvings-show-explicit-copulation.html

2. O'Connor, Roisin. "William Shakespeare was undeniably bisexual, researchers claim." *The Independent*. Accessed: June 4, 2021. https://www.independent.co.uk/arts-entertainment/books/news/shakespeare-bisexual-sexuality-evidence-plays-a9684056.html

3. Markham, Myles. "What Does the Bible Say About Homosexuality?" The Human Rights Campaign. Accessed June 4, 2021. https://www.hrc.org/resources/what-does-the-bible-say-about-homosexuality

4. Ibid.
Mack, Julie. "The 6 Bible verses on homosexuality, and differing interpretations." *Kalamazoo Gazette. Accessed: June 4, 2021.* https://www.mlive.com/news/kalamazoo/2015/08/the_7_bible_verses_on_homosexu.html
Gnuse, Robert K. "Seven Gay Texts: Biblical Passages Used to Condemn Homosexuality." *Biblical Theology Bulletin vol. 45, pp. 68–87.* https://journals.sagepub.com/doi/abs/10.1177/0146107915577097?journalCode=btba&
Horan, Daniel P. "Why the church should fight anti-transgender legislation." *National Catholic Reporter. Accessed: June 4, 2021.* https://www.ncronline.org/news/opinion/faith-seeking-understanding/why-church-should-fight-anti-transgender-legislation
Q Christian. "LGBTQ+ Theology 101." Q Christian Fellowship. Accessed: June 4, 2021. https://www.qchristian.org/resources/theology#bible

5. Oxford, Ed. "My quest to find the word 'homosexual' in the Bible." *Baptist News Global. Accessed: July 7, 2021.* https://baptistnews.com/article/my-quest-to-find-the-word-homosexual-in-the-bible/#.YOYbhy1h1Hc

6. Wikipedia. "List of animals displaying homosexual behavior: Revision history." Wikimedia Foundation. Accessed: July 7, 2021. https://en.wikipedia.org/wiki/List_of_animals_displaying_homosexual_behavior

7. PETA UK. "Gay Animals Who Prove Same-Sex Love Is Natural." People for the Ethical Treatment of Animals (PETA) Foundation. Accessed: June 13, 2021. https://www.peta.org.uk/blog/gay-animals/

Why Are Straight People Putting Their Pronouns on Zoom?

1. Ermyas, Tinbete. "Wave Of Bills To Block Trans Athletes Has No Basis In Science, Researcher Says." NPR. Accessed: June 4, 2021. https://www.npr.org/2021/03/18/978716732/wave-of-new-bills-say-trans-athletes-have-an-unfair-edge-what-does-the-science-s

2. The Trevor Project. "National Survey on LGBTQ Youth Mental Health 2021." Accessed: June 4, 2021. https://www.thetrevorproject.org/survey-2021

How Can You Use "They" for One Person If It's a Plural Word?

1. BBC News. "A brief history of gender neutral pronouns." BBC. Accessed: June 4, 2021. https://www.bbc.com/news/newsbeat-49754930

2. The International Potato Center (CIP). "Potato Facts and Figures." Accessed: June 4, 2021. https://cipotato.org/potato/potato-facts-and-figures/#:~:text=There%20are%20more%20than%204%2C000,over%20180%20wild%20potato%20species

3. The Trevor Project. "National Survey on LGBTQ Youth Mental Health 2021." Accessed: June 4, 2021. https://www.thetrevorproject.org/survey-2021

How Can I Keep My Kids Safe from Transgender and Gay People?

1. The Rape Abuse and Incest National Network (RAINN). "Victims of Sexual Violence: Statistics." RAINN. Accessed: June 4, 2021. https://www.rainn.org/statistics/victims-sexual-violence

2. PBS Newshour: Nation. "Study finds LGBTQ people much likelier to be crime victims." PBS. Accessed: June 4, 2021. https://www.pbs.org/newshour/nation/study-finds-lgbtq-people-much-likelier-to-be-crime-victims

3. The Trevor Project. "National Survey on LGBTQ Youth Mental Health 2021." Accessed: June 4, 2021. https://www.thetrevorproject.org/survey-2021

4. Alter, Charlotte. "Mike Huckabee Joked About Pretending to Be Transgender to Shower With Girls After Gym Class." TIME. Accessed: July 4, 2021. https://time.com/3905462/mike-huckabee-transgender-joke/

5. Conron, K.J. "LGBT Youth Population in the United States." The Williams Institute. Accessed: July 4, 2021. https://williamsinstitute.law.ucla.edu/wp-content/uploads/LGBT-Youth-US-Pop-Sep-2020.pdf

Conclusion: How Can I Be the Best Ally Ever?!

1. Clements, KC. "What Is Deadnaming?" Healthline. Accessed: July 4, 2021. https://www.healthline.com/health/transgender/deadnaming

2. Funders for LGBTQ Issues. "People of Color." Funders for LGBTQ Issues. Accessed: June 4, 2021. https://lgbtfunders.org/resources/issues/people-of-color/

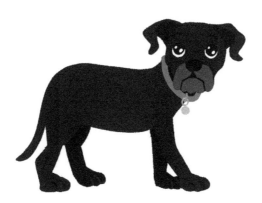

AFTERWORD

By: Peter Dawson, aka Fiona's Dad

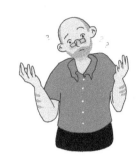

I never thought that a flippant, perhaps ill-advised remark (see Chapter 11) made to my then late-teenaged elder daughter would eventually result in a title for a book to be written from Texas more than 25 years later! We were on a family vacation at the time and wine had been taken—legal for over 18s in the UK—but Fiona's subsequent admission to her sister that she thought that she might be greedy goes unmentioned!

Having worked as a family physician for more than 30 years and subsequently for HM Courts and Tribunals service I am aware of the huge shift in public opinion and attitudes regarding sexual behaviour. In the UK in 1967, sex between two men over 21 and in private was decriminalised but it wasn't until 2000 that the age of consent of 16 was standardised for both same-sex and opposite-sex relationships. This trend of increasing social liberalisation in the UK has largely taken place over the last 30 years and has been backed by legislation, with same-sex couples being granted equal rights of adoption in 2002, gross indecency being removed as an offence in 2003, the introduction of civil partnerships in 2004, the banning of discrimination on the basis of sexual orientation in 2007, gender reassignment added as a protected characteristic in equality legislation in 2010, and the legalisation of Gay marriage in England, Wales, and Scotland in 2014. It is likely that

these changes in legislation have had a powerful influence on many people's views. More worryingly in the UK, however, over the last few years there has been a steep rise in the number of recorded homophobic hate crimes though it is not clear whether this represents a true rise in the incidence of hate crimes and/or increased confidence in reporting such incidents. Gay marriage is now legal in 29 countries across the world though same-sex relationships remain punishable by death in some Middle Eastern and African states. Naturally I am viewing matters from a UK perspective though I believe that similar, more liberalistic social trends have taken place in the USA over a similar time period; also, in much of Western Europe.

So, what does this book tell us? Fiona has a long track record of identifying areas of discrimination and injustice where people have been marginalised, unrecognised, and unheard and a brief look at her bio will confirm this. In this slim, well-written volume, 21 questions are asked and answered in a concise but amusing manner. Some answers provide helpful explanations for the relatively uninformed such as me; others act as reminders, not to make assumptions but to politely ask, listen to, and hear the answers. And then there are some others, more controversial, thought-provoking, and inviting debate. Acknowledging one's own prejudices and lack of knowledge is a key to gaining a greater appreciation and understanding of other people's views and difficulties they may experience on a daily basis. Social change occurs slowly and may take many years; and, I believe, that change needs to be backed by appropriate legislation. Before that can

happen, people need to be receptive and informed and I trust that this book will play its part in that process.

Are bisexuals greedy? Possibly, but probably no more so than the rest of us who wish to lead interesting, happy, and fulfilled lives, surrounded by the love and support of our friends and family.

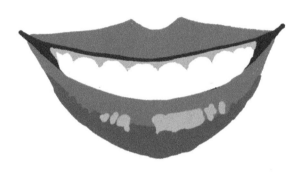

ABOUT THE AUTHOR

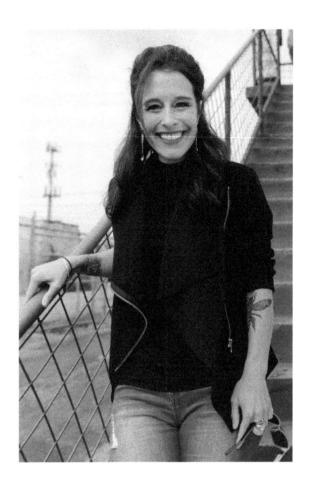

Fiona Dawson is an Emmy®-nominated and award-winning filmmaker, speaker, and author. She is a passionate believer in the power of media to educate, entertain, and inspire. With her genuine and warm heart, people describe her as the bisexual, female version of Mr. Rogers. Your Auntie Fiona.

In 1998, at the age of 21 years and before having an email address let alone a social media account, Fiona left her native home of the UK and volunteered for over six months in Bangladesh teaching English to Mande tribal people. Then, following a year of teaching at the Cambridge School in Portugal, she married her American love, emigrated to the US in 2000, and starting working for charities helping children and adults living with HIV/AIDS and survivors of domestic and sexual violence in Houston, Texas. In 2004, Fiona divorced her husband and came flying out the closet as a lesbian.

Fiona's gay visibility and advocacy earned her the election as Houston's Female Grand Marshal for the 2009 LGBT Pride Parade. She has served on the National Board of Directors of the Human Rights Campaign (HRC) and on the Board of Directors for NLGJA - The Association of LGBTQ Journalists. Fiona spent several years working in corporate social responsibility before starting her own company and moving to New York in 2011 to develop her media career.

In 2012 Fiona came out as bisexual and unrelatedly started the *TransMilitary* project to elevate the stories of active-duty transgender service members who were still banned from the US military. Following the success of the Emmy®-nominated short film *Transgender, at War and in Love* she directed and produced for *The New York Times* in 2015, Fiona was honored by The White House as an LGBT Artist Champion of Change. The film won *The White House News Photographers Association's Best Documentary*, was nominated for a GLAAD Award in the Outstanding Digital Journalism–Multimedia category, and was a nominee for Outstanding Short Documentary in the 37th Annual News & Documentary Emmy® Awards.

The feature length documentary *TransMilitary*, which Fiona codirected with SideXSide Studios' director Gabe Silverman and producer Jamie Coughlin, premiered at South by Southwest (SXSW) 2018 and won the *Best Feature Documentary Audience Award*. Following a string of festival awards, *TransMilitary* was privately screened at an event hosted in partnership with GLAAD, Logo, and The Pritzker Military Museum & Library at the US Capitol Visitor Center, with the Speaker of the House and other lawmakers present. The film made its television broadcast debut on Viacom's Logo TV in 2018 and is now available on a variety of well-known streaming platforms.

In 2020 Fiona came home to Texas, making Austin her long-term digs. As Founder and Executive Producer of Free Lion Productions, Fiona continues her work building inclusion, speaking truth, and producing kindness with a range of media production. She is working on an unscripted series that within a climate of adversity, Fiona journeys to uncover positive stories of kindness and courage from the LGBTQIA+ community, showing people are way more united than they know. The series's proof-of-concept episode premiered at Geena Davis's Bentonville Film Festival 2021, winning the Jury Award. Fiona is on a mission to decolonize the worldview of gender and sexuality with humor and ease.

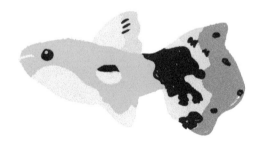

About the Illustrator

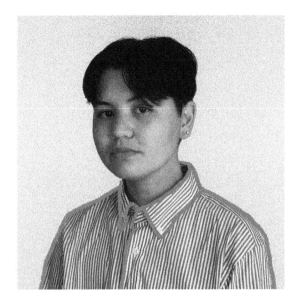

Syd Cordoba is a nonbinary artist who specializes in illustration and 2D animation. Syd's work revolves around their own personal experiences, dreams, existentialism, and of course, being queer!

Oftentimes, you can find Syd applying their skills in community-driven efforts within Richmond, Virginia, such as painting community fridges or designing visual material for local organizations and businesses.

Syd's practice is constantly teaching them new things, and sometimes challenges them in unexpected ways. They prioritize projects that have the potential to expand their knowledge about how their art can open up conversations, educate, and empower others.

WORK WITH FIONA

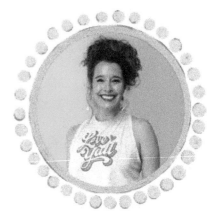

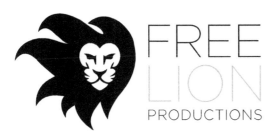

FREELIONPRODUCTIONS.COM

FIONA DAWSON (SHE/HER)
FOUNDER & DIRECTOR
HELLO@FREELIONPRODUCTIONS.COM

Building Inclusion.

WE DELIVER:
- ♥ Unscripted Film Production
- ♥ Animated Explainer Videos
- ♥ Speaking Engagements

YOU GAIN:
- ♥ Boosted talent attraction and retention.
- ♥ Enhanced culture of inclusion and belonging.
- ♥ Customized, evergreen, multi-purpose content that builds empathy.

DIFFERENTIATORS:
- ♥ Center on people's values, experience, and aspirations.
- ♥ Merge award-winning filmmaking with corporate, international, DEIBA (diversity, equity, inclusion, belonging, and accessibility) expertise.
- ♥ Outshine traditional production studio budgets.

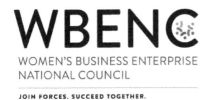

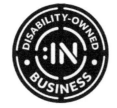

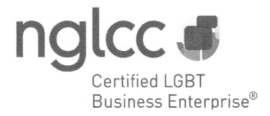

CORPORATE DEIBA EXPERTS & EMMY®-NOMINATED AND AWARD-WINNING FILMMAKERS

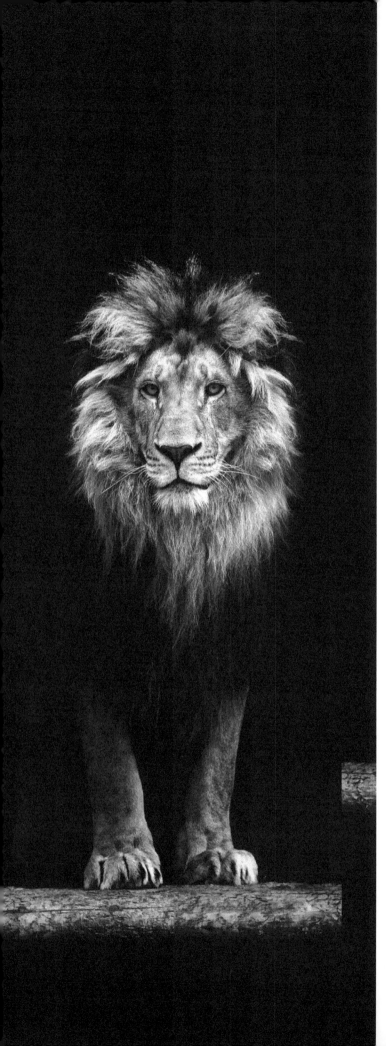

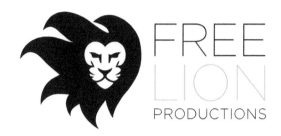

Free Lion Productions is a multi-media production company building inclusion, sharing truth, and producing kindness.

♥

VISION STATEMENT

We envision a day when all people are treated with equitable rights, equitable respect, and equitable responsibility.

♥

CORE VALUES

Gratitude · Mindfulness
Integrity · Joy · Courage

♥

MISSION STATEMENT

We are on a mission to decolonize the worldview of gender and sexuality with humor and ease.

freelionproductions.com

Printed in the USA
CPSIA information can be obtained
at www.ICGtesting.com
CBHW061130250624
10629CB00027B/1199